Prader-Willi Syndrome

Prader-Willi Syndrome

How Parents and Professionals
Struggled and Coped
and Made Genetic History

JOHN HERNANDEZ-STORR

ISBN-13: 9780997178302
ISBN-10: 0997178302

To my mother, Carol, my first and biggest fan
And to Naomi, without whom there would be no book

Table of Contents

Introduction

My daughter Naomi seemed normal at first, with the proper number of fingers and toes, a full head of black hair, and cheeks the color of tomato soup. But she slept a lot, even for a newborn. She didn't cry. She didn't nurse much.

The medical diagnosis was hypotonia, meaning low muscle tone. A young doctor told us it sometimes resolved on its own. After four days in the hospital, our pediatrician let us go home for Christmas, but she wanted us back in her office the next day.

At the December 26, 2002 appointment, Naomi hung from the pediatrician's hand like cooked spaghetti. The pediatrician sent us back to the hospital, Cedars-Sinai, in Los Angeles. I felt like I had been teleported to a barren mountaintop. Specialists came in and out of the hospital room, and I waited to see which would show us the way down the mountain. Infectious disease? Muscle disorder? Metabolic disorder? Neurology? Genetics?

I heard the term "Prader-Willi" for the first time from the geneticist. I googled it. The initial stage admittedly described Naomi: low muscle tone, sleepy baby, poor feeder. Then it got weird. Somewhere around two to four years of age these kids' appetites get locked into the "on" position. If not controlled by others, they eat so much and get so obese that they die in their teens or twenties. And there are behavioral problems, emotional problems, medical problems. Hormone deficiencies, infertility, stubbornness, temper tantrums.

No thanks! It was a random genetic error that happened only in about one in fifteen thousand births, so I was pretty sure that roulette ball would land on some other poor family. But the genetic test for Prader-Willi syndrome came back positive.

I looked for a loophole. I said to a doctor: "But… she could still be a mother some day, couldn't she? Couldn't you give her hormone injections so she would be fertile?"

The doctor looked dubious. "She would eat the baby's food."

I slumped in my chair in the hospital room. I ached for the girl I'd lost—the one who would go to college, get married, have children. Later that day another doctor saw me feeling sorry for myself and stared at me for a few moments, as if trying to pick his next words carefully. Finally he said, "At least she's going to walk and talk," and turned away.

That same day I googled "Prader-Willi association" and found PWSA (USA), located in Florida. They put us in touch with a local Prader-Willi parent, who called us that evening.

She had a son with PWS who was four years old. She assured us that her son was wonderful. She said not to go by the information we found on the web, that much of it was old. Today there was a treatment—growth hormone—that improved muscle tone. And there were early interventions: physical therapy, speech therapy, occupational therapy. No one could predict Naomi's future, but there was much hope that her life would be a good one.

A few weeks later we met with the geneticist, Rena Falk. All I remember is what happened at the end.

I said, "Do you have any more information on the syndrome? Something written?"

Falk's young assistant jumped up and pulled a book off a shelf. I saw Falk reach to intercept it, but she was too slow.

The cover was a faded blue-green with big black letters spelling out "Management of Prader-Willi Syndrome." I opened it and read the foreword, by a doctor named Hans Zellweger.

> I have had a major interest in Prader-Willi syndrome for over 30 years and, having dealt with many patients, have reached the conclusion that PWS is one of the two most grave ailments I have encountered—the other being Huntington's Disease. Anyone who has witnessed the mood swings and the relentless, progressive, intellectual, and physical deterioration associated with HD would agree beyond a doubt that it is a devastating condition. PWS is an equally devastating birth

defect that characteristically presents major problems from birth.

My chest constricted. The words started to float around on the page. I blinked and read on.

Parents, usually unable to manage diets, food-seeking activities, and bizarre behavior, become distraught and emotionally drained. Family systems deteriorate and life becomes hell for all concerned. In my experience, parents of PWS children come to the physician's office in great distress and total despair more often than parents of children with any other birth defect.

I stopped reading. I shut the book and handed it back. I felt sorry for those families who'd suffered so much in the past. It was going to be a lot better for Naomi.

For the next six years I maintained that attitude. Naomi was slow to develop—crawling at twelve months, using single words at fourteen months, walking at twenty-four months—but she did indeed become a walker and a talker, helped along by the growth hormone shots she began getting at two months of age. I kept waiting for her appetite to burst onto the scene like the shark in *Jaws*, but what happened was subtler. When she ate, her eyes would close or roll back in her head. Sometimes it almost seemed she was falling asleep, but her mouth kept working. She savored her mushy little baby hot dogs or pureed vegetables like someone tasting ice cream after a weeklong fast. When she ate, she maintained complete focus on her food. She did not take questions. She ate, and that was all.

Then—kindergarten. We thought we were prepared. She'd had two years of special needs preschool and now she would enter a regular public elementary school kindergarten class. The kindergarten teacher explained that the children would experience tremendous growth, as they learned to follow directions, socialize with their peers, and learn together. They would get with the program.

Naomi did not get with the program. She did not want to be told when to stop reading, when to stop playing on the playground, when to sit down and listen to a story. She would refuse to move. She would flop on the playground's asphalt instead of coming back to the classroom. She started peeing in her pants, even though she'd been toilet trained for a couple of years. She sometimes scratched, hit, or kicked when the staff tried to physically redirect her.

I made my second call to the national Prader-Willi association in Florida, and was put in touch with a counselor. I told him about Naomi's problems, her obstinacy, her refusal to participate.

He chuckled. He said her obstinacy sounded a lot like the adults with PWS who were on the association's advisory board.

After I got off the phone, I thought back to what Zellweger had written and what the counselor had just told me. Had I been living under a delusion the past six years? Were the behavior problems of PWS just as bad as they'd always been? Was it still a special hell for families?

I'd been thinking about writing a book about PWS, and now I decided to go ahead with it. I'd been a history major in college, and now history had a new urgency. I wanted to know about families who'd come before me. How had they handled their children with PWS from childhood into adulthood? Had they made good lives for them? I wanted to know the medical and scientific history of PWS: What had been learned about this odd syndrome? Why did it happen? What could be done about it?

I got to know the founding families of the national association, PWSA (USA), and got their permission to write about their children's lives. I got to know some of the key scientists who had unraveled the genetic mystery of PWS, and some of the professionals who had figured out treatments. This book is my answer to the questions I posed back in 2009.

Part I

Joining the Struggle

One

PRADER-WHATEVER

"Curtis has Prader-Willi syndrome."

Fausta and Gene Deterling stared at Dr. Bresnan. For five months, since Curtis's birth on March 28, 1971, the doctors had offered only vagueness; the sudden specificity was unnerving.

"What does that mean?" Gene asked.

Bresnan frowned, and his eyes moved around the room. "Some Swiss doctors described it. The babies are born just like Curtis—very weak muscles, they can hardly cry or suck. The boys have underdeveloped testes, like Curtis. They do eventually walk and talk. But when they get about two years old, they become obese."

Gene and Fausta blinked at each other. Obese? Their floppy little guy with hardly any appetite?

"They're also short, with small hands and feet. And they're not a hundred percent mentally. They get more and more obese. He'll get so heavy his organs will fail. He probably won't make it past his teens or at best his twenties."

Gene stared at him. He was an engineer and a manager, a problem solver. "Can't we do something?"

Bresnan shook his head. "You'll want to think about placing him with an institution."

As they drove away from Boston Children's Hospital, back to their home in Natick, they stared at the landscape. Why did everything look the same when nothing would ever be the same? But by the time they reached their home, a little thought had fluttered between them: what if Bresnan was mistaken? There was no lab test for this weird syndrome. Weak muscles. Underdeveloped genitals. Couldn't that be any number of things? Sara and Evan, their older children, would be home from school soon. Gene had to get back to work. Curtis needed a bottle. Away from the hospital, the doctor's words lost some of their power.

One thing was clear: putting Curtis in an institution was not an option. They would not give up their baby. They were not some green couple. Their bond was strong; it had not taken them long to see the "ever after" in each other's eyes. Gene had proposed to Fausta six weeks after their first proper date, and they'd married three months after that.

Fausta had been given her unusual name—from Empress Fausta, wife of Constantine the Great—by her mother. People chronically mispronounced Fausta's name, which annoyed her. It wasn't pronounced like Goethe's Faust; it was pronounced "FAW-stuh." It amused Gene when he would introduce himself and his wife to people, and they would grab his hand and say, "How do you do, Foster?" and turn to his wife and say, "Nice to meet you, Jean."

Their shared sense of humor helped them through the bumps of early married life—the "do you really love me?" times. Sara came along in 1961 and Evan two years later. Eventually it seemed to Gene and Fausta that they'd been born married. When Fausta became pregnant with Curtis, eight years after Evan was born, it was a surprise, but one the whole family welcomed.

Sara was a tomboy who roamed the suburban woods and swamps collecting snakes and frogs, but Curtis brought out her nurturing instincts. She loved to sit next to her mom and watch her give Curtis his tiny bottle, even though it took a long time. Evan was a thoughtful boy who had learned to read early by studying the labels of jars and containers in the fridge. He was also a kind boy, and he liked playing with his baby brother. Fausta was a warm and competent mother who could stay home with the kids because Gene made a good living at Honeywell. Gene often helped out on the night shift, giving Curtis his bottle so Fausta could rest.

But even a well-knit family wouldn't be enough to save Curtis if Bresnan's dire prediction came true. Gene was scared for his infant son. His evening prayers often began, "God, give me courage." Fausta was scared, too. But she also wondered if her mother was right. When Fausta had told her mother about Bresnan's diagnosis, her mother had said, "Oh, doctors don't know everything. He'll probably outgrow it."

It looked like his grandmother was prophetic, as Curtis kept improving. At nine months he could finally hold up his head. He was starting to babble. When he was ten months old, Sara was watching him in his playpen and heard him say "Mama." She darted upstairs to tell Fausta that Curtis had said his first word. He'd come a long way from the feeble newborn who hardly ever cried, and when he did, made a squeak like a tiny bird. Some of his mannerisms made them laugh. He would hold his hands in front of his face, studying them and solemnly moving them about. Fausta said he was blessing them.

In March 1973, two weeks before he turned two, Curtis took his first steps. Sara and a friend were playing with him, and Curtis managed to wobble his way between them. He was delayed, but hitting all his milestones. He had also found his appetite. He had become chubby, but not remarkably so. The failure-to-thrive period was just a bad memory, and it seemed entirely possible that this Prader-Whatever business would fade away, too.

The family was moving up in the world. Around the time Curtis turned one, Gene's job moved northwest of Boston, and Gene convinced the company to pay for him to move, too. The family left Natick for Harvard, an even leafier town (despite the name, the town has no connection with Harvard University). The family loved Harvard. It was beautiful, dotted with apple orchards and riding stables. It was prosperous and cozy—the graduating high school class had just sixty students.

But like an unshakable fairy-tale curse, Bresnan's dark words followed them to their new home. Curtis went from chubby to undeniably fat. At a visit to Bresnan when Curtis was two and a half, his weight was above the ninety-seventh percentile, while his height was below the third percentile. He was a very round little boy. Fausta could hardly believe what was happening. She'd been monitoring his eating, and she was sure he wasn't getting too much food. She had raised two kids who were at normal weight. So how could Curtis be getting so fat?

It had to be the strange syndrome. Gene and Fausta felt it drape over them like a lead coat. Prader-Willi. Prader-Willi. They grieved for the boy they weren't going to have—the boy who would grow tall and strong like Gene, who would one day find his Fausta and have his own little bundles of joy and sorrow. Curtis's life would be a shorter, much more limited one, according to Bresnan. But in their fog something else was forming, something as hard and stubborn as the reality they faced. A recurring thought: there must be something we can do. But what?

Well, they could try to learn more. That would be a start. During a visit to Bresnan, they asked for more information. He let them read a short section about the syndrome from a book in his office. The doctor was glad to see that the Deterlings had accepted reality, but he was cautious about their desire to learn more. While he figured reading the short description in his book wouldn't do them any harm, he wasn't sure he wanted them to know everything in the medical literature. They might be better off ignorant. The picture of Prader-Willi syndrome that doctors had pieced together since its discovery in 1956 was a disturbing one.

Two

A Fatal Syndrome

Hans Zellweger was a tall adventuresome doctor from a patrician family in Chur, the oldest town in Switzerland. In his youth, after World War I, he had seen the horrific effects of a polio epidemic. His life goal was to understand neuromuscular disorders that affected children. He trained across Europe and worked with Albert Schweitzer in Africa. After returning to Switzerland, Zellweger became chief resident at the children's hospital in Zurich, the Kinderspital, where he started tracking cases of significant muscle weakness in infants—babies who were, in medical jargon, hypotonic, or more descriptively, floppy. He wanted to untangle the various causes.

Zellweger noticed that sometimes the floppy babies also had hormone problems. In a paper he published in 1946, he described one who had become very fat at a young age—and, in retrospect, probably had PWS. But the other case he described was thin. Zellweger had come close, but he had not yet zeroed in on PWS.

Zellweger left Zurich for Beirut in 1951. Andrea Prader, another Swiss pediatrician, became the new chief resident at the Kinderspital. Prader was ten years younger than Zellweger and had been trained by Zellweger in pediatrics. Prader's family had made a fortune in construction, but he was not interested in luxuries. He drove an old car. What he did care about was making scientific discoveries.

Prader picked up Zellweger's floppy baby project, and he spotted a unique pattern in a patient named Albert, whom he had first seen with Zellweger: floppy at birth, underdeveloped genitals, fat by around two years old, short, with small hands and feet, and mentally retarded. Prader, in collaboration with Heinrich Willi, the head of the newborn nursery, and Alexis Labhart, an endocrinologist in private practice, identified eight other cases, all younger than Albert. Four were boys, four were girls. They published their paper in 1956, with Prader as the first author. (Labhart was eventually dropped from the name of the syndrome, but Prader always insisted on recognizing Labhart's role, and Willi's, too.)

Discovering the syndrome was a huge achievement, although it was not recognized as such at the time. The paper was published in a small Swiss journal, in German. It was no more than a brief description. Neither Prader, nor Labhart, nor Willi had any idea what caused the syndrome, or how to treat it. Five years after the paper was published, Albert died at twenty-eight from the complications of years of obesity.

In the 1960s, other doctors began to investigate. The most immediate question was what was causing the patients to get so fat? Two English doctors thought it was a metabolic problem. But the majority view in the 1960s was simpler: people with PWS were just eating too much. They were driven to overeat, and their appetites lacked an "off switch." The descriptions in the medical articles were lurid. Two teen-age boys habitually searched garbage cans for food. Another boy would eat the cattle feed from his father's farm. A sixteen-year-old girl would sneak into the refrigerator at night and eat raw sausage.

Prader and Willi had at least one positive thing to report, in a follow-up paper published in 1963. They described their PWS patients as good-natured. But over the next few years, a different picture emerged.

After eight years in Beirut, Hans Zellweger moved one more time, to the University of Iowa, in 1959. He began diagnosing Prader-Willi syndrome in his patients, and by the late 1960s he had fourteen cases, enough to make some general observations. In 1969 he wrote that they had "a deficient control of their emotions." He continued: "They show exuberant feelings of joy and pleasure. They go almost into rapture when their nurse or doctor appears in the morning. They hug them and express their sympathy in words and deeds without the slightest inhibition. On the other hand, they can be extremely stubborn and fully inaccessible to any kind of exhortations. If they do not want to be examined, for instance, there is little chance that one can persuade them to comply. Temper tantrums are not rare in these children."

In 1972, a review of PWS was published in *The Journal of Pediatrics*, a publication widely read by pediatricians. The authors surveyed thirty-two cases of PWS—the most ever assembled. They saw their patients as affectionate until about three years of age, with temper tantrums and stubbornness coming in after that. By late adolescence and adulthood it was even worse: "With limited provocation, sudden acts of violence and displays of temper were common, as were states of depression."

Small wonder that Curtis's doctor was cautious about exposing Gene and Fausta Deterling to the medical literature. The message there for parents was: your child will inevitably become quite obese and an ever-worsening behavior problem. And doctors had noticed other problems. Eye problems—and indeed, Curtis was born with crossed eyes, which were partially corrected by surgery. Speech defects. Excessive daytime sleepiness. And as the children aged, scoliosis—sideways curvature of the spine—which in more severe cases was painful and put the internal organs of the chest at risk.

Many families did not know what to do with children like these, and in the 1950s and 1960s a common solution was to give them up to be raised by an institution. The medical articles of the time gave brief, bland descriptions of the fates of these children. In England, an eleven-year-old girl with PWS was committed to an institution on the grounds that she was too obese and mentally retarded to be cared for in the community. Another English girl with PWS was committed at age sixteen, weighing 260 pounds. She had been stealing food, and was labeled mentally retarded. In Sweden, a baby boy with PWS was placed in a home for the mentally deficient. Cut off from his parents and siblings, he did the opposite of thrive. He didn't crawl until he was four years old, and never did learn to talk.

Other families kept their Prader-Willi children with them, but even families with resources struggled. In Boston in the early 1970s, a young man with PWS was in a precarious state. At eighteen years old, he stood four feet eleven inches tall and weighed 238 pounds. He was given amphetamines to try to curb his appetite, and tranquilizers and psychological support to try to curb his behaviors. It didn't work—a year later he had gained 25 more pounds. Because his life was in danger, he was given a drastic procedure that removed 90 percent of his small intestine. That did succeed in reducing his weight somewhat, but at the cost of chronic diarrhea and metabolic problems.

The medical literature in the early 1970s had nothing good in it for the Deterlings. Curtis was already obese and seemingly destined for a short and unhappy life. But fate was about to give the Deterlings a gift.

Three

A DRASTIC DIET

Even though Bresnan had a grim view of Curtis's future prospects, he wanted to do something to help. After seeing Curtis at his two-and-a-half-year visit, he decided that at the next visit he would refer the Deterlings to a dietitian. True to his plan, when he saw Curtis six months later, in May 1974, he sent the Deterlings to a dietitian at Boston Children's Hospital. That simple act would end up doing far more than Bresnan could have envisioned—because the dietitian he referred them to connected the Deterlings with Peggy Pipes, a dietitian in Seattle who had recently developed a plan that could save Curtis's life.

When Pipes was in high school, in Texas, she'd been impressed with a female teacher who combined nutrition and chemistry. Practical and smart, Pipes thought. She got a bachelor of science in food and nutrition from Texas Tech, then went to New York City for an internship. She discovered how much she liked working with babies, and from then on her focus was pediatric nutrition.

Over the next two decades Pipes worked and collected two master's degrees. In 1968 she visited a friend in Seattle, at the Child Development and Mental Retardation Clinic affiliated with the University of Washington. The clinic was looking for a nutritionist, and Pipes asked, "Will you consider me?" She would stay for 28 years.

The Seattle clinic and a few others like it were pioneering clinics for kids with disabilities, set up during the Kennedy administration. At the Seattle clinic, Pipes met Vanja Holm, a diminutive doctor with the lilting accent of her home country of Sweden. Holm was born north of the Arctic Circle, and got her medical degree in Stockholm. There, she met and fell in love with an American studying economics. They were married in the early 1950s, and together they moved back to his native Seattle, where they had two children. Holm focused on kids with handicaps, such as cerebral palsy and Down syndrome. It took her longer to become aware of Prader-Willi syndrome. In 1969 she began reading up on the syndrome and realized that she already had a few cases at the clinic.

That year a young boy named Russell Iverson was referred to the clinic with a diagnosis of Prader-Willi syndrome. He was eighteen months old and not yet overweight. Holm was excited: here was a chance to try to prevent a Prader-Willi child from becoming obese. She told Peggy Pipes to work with Russell and his mom. Pipes carefully instructed the mom on an appropriate diet for a child of Russell's age. But one year later Russell was obese. He'd gone from the twenty-fifth to the ninety-seventh percentile in weight.

What went wrong? Russell's mom insisted that her son was not eating more than Pipes prescribed. Pipes wanted to see for herself. She admitted Russell and his mother to a residential facility at the clinic for three weeks. Russell was put on a stringent diet of 800 calories per day and weighed regularly. Pipes and the other workers watched him through one-way mirrors to check that he wasn't sneaking food.

The result: Russell lost more than a pound—proof that a child with PWS could lose weight. Pipes's careful measurements and calculations also showed that Russell needed noticeably fewer calories than a normal child. He and his mom went back home and, continuing the diet for three months, got his weight back down to the ninetieth percentile. Energized, Pipes developed a home program and used it successfully on three other young boys with PWS.

Pipes and Holm published their findings in the *Journal of the American Dietetic Association* in 1973. These two women, a Texan and a Swede, did what a decade and a half of male doctors had failed to do: fend off the deadly obesity of Prader-Willi syndrome. They also made clear just what parents of kids with the syndrome were up against. Pipes's careful measurements showed that children with PWS needed on average just 60 percent of the calories of normal kids; anything more than that, and they would gain weight. Pipes and Holm had just ended the medical debate of the 1960s, when doctors wondered if kids with PWS were so fat because of metabolism or appetite. The answer was, both.

This posed a new question: was this some cruel joke of nature? To combine a sluggish metabolism with a raging appetite? And it came on top of the other irony of the syndrome: that the deadly appetite emerged only gradually, and after an initial phase of undereating, guaranteeing that parents would be celebrating rather than guarding against their child's newfound interest in food. No wonder Hans Zellweger had been so pessimistic. What chance did families have, not knowing what they were dealing with?

At least parents had some chance now, thanks to Peggy Pipes and Vanja Holm. When word spread that a dietitian at the Seattle clinic had had success in controlling the weight of a child with PWS, more and more children with the syndrome found their way to the clinic. And the more patients they saw, the more Pipes and Holm learned. They heard all about the unusual food behaviors of these children—how they were preoccupied with food, worrying whether there would be enough and asking repeatedly about their next meal. How they would creep quietly from their beds at night to sneak food. How they would grab and gobble up sticks of butter from the dinner table. How they would slip over to their pets' food bowls and eat the dog or cat food.

They also heard how unhelpful professionals could be. How one mother pleaded for a calorie-restricted diet when she left her two-year-old at a community hospital and returned two hours later to find seven popsicle sticks in the wastebasket.

How a preschool teacher said she would follow the diet but in fact felt the mother was exaggerating and secretly gave the child extra snacks.

Pipes and Holm realized that if parents were going to successfully shepherd their ravenous kids through a world laced with food, they needed more than just a diet. Their solution was drastic: complete environmental control of food. At home, food had to be hidden and locked up. Food given to a child with PWS had to be carefully measured and tracked. Every family member had to buy into the plan. And parents would have to explain the situation to teachers and other parents, who likely would view these actions as cruel and unnecessary.

Pipes and Holm were saying that instead of trying to "fix" kids with PWS—giving them amphetamines, or tranquilizers, or psychotherapy, or intestinal surgery—the environment around the kids needed to be fixed. What these kids needed was a protective buffer between themselves and the world.

And that buffer was not just physical, but psychological. They told parents to be positive with their children, not negative. Praise them for looking better after they lost weight—they seemed highly motivated by praise. And if a child somehow got extra food, by sneaking or gorging, don't berate or shame the child, but simply make a calorie adjustment.

Pipes and Holm got crucial help from the mothers, especially Shirley Neason, mother of Pipes's second patient, Daniel. It was Shirley who came up with the idea of locking the refrigerator and making food completely inaccessible. Shirley, as well as Russell's mother, also gave Pipes important data when for months they meticulously measured and logged every single thing their sons ate.

Holm and Pipes began to attract attention. A reporter at the *The Seattle Daily Times* found out about their work with PWS, and interviewed Holm for a story. Some days later a Tacoma paper called Holm, and then a San Francisco paper. Holm was learning that newspaper editors read each other's papers to get ideas. Then the story went national. The Associated Press picked it up and wrote an article that was published in many papers around the United States in the summer of 1975. The articles would generally appear in the Sunday editions, and on Mondays Holm got used to having a long list of phone calls to return, as colleagues around the country excitedly called to report having seen her name in the paper.

The highlight for Holm came when *Newsweek* ran an article on her and the clinic in October 1975. The article filled two-thirds of a page and featured a large picture of Holm, in a wide-lapel shirt, smiling beatifically at a young boy with PWS, who was gazing happily at a lunchbox. After the *Newsweek* article came an article in *Today's Health*, a magazine for doctors' offices that specialized in medical drama, and then an article in *Good Housekeeping*.

Holm was pleased that all the articles described the syndrome fairly accurately and mentioned the work of her clinic. But she was not so pleased to discover what the journalists thought about the syndrome.

The Associated Press called PWS "rare and horrifying." *Newsweek* labeled it "bizarre" and the kids' appetites "monstrous."

Good Housekeeping referred to it as "frightening and baffling." *Today's Health* called Holm and Pipes's work "quixotic." The author of the *Today's Health* article, Carolyn See, was a freelance journalist who had just published a piece on anorexia nervosa, the disease of dangerous undereating, in the previous month's issue. Now her editors were sending her to Seattle to write a sort of counterpoint on this strange new disease of overeating. See was a practitioner of "new journalism"—Tom Wolfe style—parachuting in with no preconceptions and soaking it all up.

"It's desperately hard for parents of these children," See wrote. To keep their kids alive, they had to stand constant guard over all food. Worse, the kids—especially as they got older—would engage in ghastly tantrums. It was an endless grind. And even a short break was nearly impossible. "They can't, for instance, go to the movies, because of buttered popcorn, Jujubees, Raisinets, and the ensuing tantrum in the lobby. They can't—God forbid!—go out to a restaurant. And if they go by themselves, leaving the child with a sitter, typically the child begs food, and failing his demands, indulges in yet another extended tantrum. An alternate decision, to leave the child with his siblings, may not be altogether safe. One young boy, on being denied food by his brother, chased him around the house with a knife."

Families broke under the pressure. See got to know a seventeen-year-old named Lynda, whose parents' marriage had fractured. Before the divorce, Lynda's mom was vigilant, and Lynda lost a good deal of weight. But after the divorce, her mom lost control, and Lynda, who was just five feet one inch tall, weighed 233 pounds. Lynda's mom refused to meet with Peggy Pipes. She was afraid of what Pipes would say. Instead Lynda's mom met with the clinic's kindly educator, who tried to convince her to lock up the food.

But things had gone too far, and Lynda's mom was too afraid to do it. "You don't know how it would be! The howls she'd put up! Oh, it's a roar, I'll tell you. I'm really frightened of her when she screams at me like that. She's bigger than I am, you know, twice as big. And the noise she makes! The last time we had a fight over food she went out on the front porch, right out in the street, and simply bellowed."

This was the paradox of Prader-Willi syndrome in the mid-1970s. On the one hand, Peggy Pipes and Vanja Holm's common-sense approach had wiped away the fatalism—the assumption that, as they put it, "gross obesity is the inevitable fate of these children." They had given parents a realistic, though demanding, program to keep their children's weight in check. On the other hand, Carolyn See and the other journalists were not incorrect in portraying PWS as a soul-crushing struggle for many families. Hans Zellweger's gloomy description of the disorder was largely accurate.

Pipes and Holm's discoveries were an important start, but they were not a complete program for dealing with the disorder. And their work was spreading too slowly from their Seattle base to help many of the families sinking from the weight of Prader-Willi.

Four

Parents Band Together

In early 1974 Gene Deterling was restless. Curtis was plumping up rapidly, and nothing Gene and Fausta did seemed to help. They had not yet been referred to a dietitian; they had not yet heard of Peggy Pipes. The persistent thought—*there must be something we can do*—nagged at Gene. He began thinking of other families dealing with Prader-Willi syndrome. What was it like for them? Were they all struggling, too? Had some of them figured out something he didn't know?

Gene thought perhaps he and Fausta could start an organization. That way parents could share their knowledge, share their resources, support each other, and help all their kids. At the next appointment with Bresnan in May 1974, Gene told him his idea.

That was the same doctor's appointment when Bresnan finally referred the Deterlings to the dietitian in Boston who told them about Pipes and Holm's breakthrough. Gene and

Fausta were delighted: here were professionals who had actually come up with a helpful plan.

Fausta set about measuring and monitoring Curtis's food. Over the following months, they watched Curtis's weight gain slow, stop, and go into reverse. Starting at an obese 47 pounds in spring 1974, Curtis actually lost 5 pounds over the next year and a half while growing taller. It felt like a miracle. Curtis was no longer their doomed child.

Now Gene knew exactly who to contact about his idea for an organization. In November 1974 he wrote to Peggy Pipes. She wrote back, encouraging him to follow through and giving him the name of a parent in the Seattle area who could help him: Shirley Neason. Shirley was known as "Tough Lady" around the Seattle PWS clinic for her success in controlling her son's weight. Shirley also had a thoughtfulness and kindness that impressed the clinic staff, including Pipes.

Gene and Fausta wrote Shirley, proposing that they work together to start a Prader-Willi organization for parents and interested professionals like Holm and Pipes. Soon Gene and Shirley were talking on the phone. They were surprised at how much they had in common. Both marriages had quickly produced a boy and a girl two years apart, and then after an eight-year gap, a third and final child, a boy with Prader-Willi syndrome. Both Gene and T. G., Shirley's husband, had managerial positions at leading companies—Gene at Honeywell, T. G. at Boeing.

Gene proposed that Shirley edit a newsletter while he handle the organization. Shirley accepted. She was already used to volunteering; this would be a chance to continue serving others and learn more about the syndrome. She had a manual Royal typewriter, so she had the basic tool to put together a newsletter.

In summer 1975 all five Deterlings got in a motor home and drove from Harvard to Seattle to spend a couple of days with the Neasons. Curtis was four years old and loved vehicles, so spending all that time in a motor home was a big thrill.

The couples shared stories of how the words "Prader-Willi syndrome" had come into their lives. The Neasons were surprised that Curtis had been diagnosed at just five months of age, before he'd even become obese. Daniel had been nearly three years old, and quite fat, when the Neasons got the diagnosis at the University of Washington hospital.

Like the Deterlings, the Neasons had initially been told that there was nothing they could do to save Daniel from an early death from obesity. They had been told to just enjoy him as he was. It was nearly a year after Daniel's initial diagnosis when Peggy Pipes reached out to them, after her success with her first child with PWS. Most exciting for the Deterlings was the chance they had to see a well-managed child with PWS who was four years older than Curtis. Daniel was a talkative, curious boy. He liked to read the encyclopedia, going from article to article. He attended his local public school and was in a regular classroom. He did have a hard time socializing with his peers, who sensed his differences. But overall Daniel seemed happy in school and was doing enough to get by academically.

Shirley and Gene split off from the others to make a stop at the Seattle clinic. They met with Peggy Pipes in a conference room and had the first face-to-face meeting of the brand new organization, which they called Prader-Willi Syndrome Parents and Friends (it would be renamed Prader-Willi Syndrome Association two years later). Peggy Pipes was impressed by Gene's organizational skills. He wanted the newsletter, which he named *The Gathered View*, to come out every two months, and for the first issue to come out that summer.

Gene and Shirley returned to the Neasons' house, and soon it was time to say good-bye. It was exciting for Gene and Fausta to make contact with a family in many ways their mirror image. Daniel, like Curtis, had his weight under control and a world of possibilities ahead of him. With Shirley keeping watch over him, he was clearing a trail that Curtis might happily follow.

Five

Shirley Rising

The first issue of *The Gathered View* came out in July 1975 and was mailed to all ten members of the new organization. Shirley gave her recipe for low-calorie lemonade. Gene and Fausta shared a list of exercises they did with Curtis. Gene wrote about Curtis's first four years of life and asked other parents to write about their children. Peggy Pipes and Vanja Holm described their plan for weight control.

During the next year, 1976, membership climbed steadily, from 51 in January to 180 by November, with members in thirty-three states. Gene had imagined a nationwide organization, but reality outran his dreams, and by the end of the year there were also members from England, Canada, Australia, and West Germany.

Parents reported problems that had never been written up in any medical article. In the January 1976 newsletter, Judith Gelb wrote from Australia to say that her daughter had a bad habit of picking at scratches on her skin until they bled. She wondered if other children had similar habits. Shirley responded that Daniel also picked his skin. In the following newsletters, other parents reported that their children picked their skin. Soon the doctors caught on and realized that skin picking was, oddly enough, another hallmark of PWS.

Other issues discussed by parents in the first two years of the newsletters included low-calorie cooking, ways to promote physical development, whether schools should use food for behavior modification, whether some children had stronger food drives than others, gastric surgery, residential facilities for teens and adults, work programs for adults, how to start a local parents' group, and bed-wetting. Gene and Fausta were delighted. The newsletter had become the venue for a nationwide—worldwide—conversation about how to deal with Prader-Willi syndrome.

As the conversation swirled, Shirley had more and more to say. She was reluctant at first—she wrote in an early issue that she "had no journalism training and welcomed advice." But she had a feeling for what her readers wanted and needed. She gave them recipes, book reviews, and summaries of presentations by experts at the Seattle clinic.

Shirley became a reporter, writing about the pioneering summer camp and residential facility for people with PWS, run by Margo Thornley in the Seattle area. She began describing things she was doing that seemed to help Daniel. She wrote about his skin picking: "I treat the area he picks with baby oil or ointment. We also tell him that it's his skin and he can pick at it if he wants to, but that it's very unpleasant and we don't like it." In the January 1977 issue, she printed a note she had written for Daniel's teacher about the specific issues of children with PWS. Her introduction was modest: "Another Prader-Willi mother read my note and asked for a copy for her child's teacher. As a result, I decided to print it in case other parents might have some use for it."

From observing Daniel and other children with PWS, Shirley drew a psychological portrait:

Distractibility: He is easily distracted by what those around him are doing and needs guidance to refocus.

Difficulty with self-correction: When he gets on the wrong track, he often can't correct himself without guidance.

Lacks social skills: He has difficulty relating appropriately to peers. He needs to be taught what to do.

Needs well-defined limits: He functions best when an adult maintains clear limits. He cannot handle as much independence as a normal child.

Shirley also got involved in an ambitious group project to write a comprehensive handbook for parents. Vanja Holm and other staff at the Seattle clinic had encouraged a group of mothers to carry out the project. But after a year of thinking about it and doing some writing, the others fell away.

Shirley decided to carry forward on her own, and after much effort she had a complete draft. Holm and Pipes revised the chapters on the description of the syndrome and weight control. And it was done.

Gene had agreed to have the association publish it, but they needed funds. The money came from a memorial fund for an eighteen-year-old with PWS who had just died; his parents hoped that the handbook would help other children avoid their child's fate.

Shirley could finally write "It's Here!" in the July 1978 newsletter. Copies began to be distributed around the country and the world. Australians had formed their own Prader-Willi association and were selling the handbook. A group in England passed a single copy of the handbook among themselves. A doctor in Puerto Rico translated a synopsis of it into Spanish. Within six months, 370 of the 500 copies were sold, and within a year it had to be reprinted. Gene hailed the handbook as a "superb accomplishment." It was helpful, realistic, and encouraging. Shirley urged parents, "Accept your child as he is, not as you wished at one time that he would be." She told them to become activists for their kids, even if that meant agitating for changes in the law regarding services and education for people with handicaps.

On the key issue of dealing with temper tantrums, she advised prevention through adequate diet, rest, and exercise, and keeping the child informed of upcoming plans to avoid sudden disruption or disappointment. She suggested parents try to increase their child's independence: "The more he can do without interference from others, the less occasion for conflict." And she suggested acceptance of minor quirks: "Be tolerant of his idiosyncrasies rather than trying to mold him into conformity." But if a tantrum did occur, "It is advisable to make sure the child does not achieve his desired goal."

She was understanding of the difficulties of dealing with overeating and obesity: "If, however, after having done your best to control his weight, your child still becomes obese, don't ruin your own health worrying about it. Obesity is the natural state of a person with PWS. If you overcome it, you have won a victory against great odds; if you do not overcome it, you have still done a good thing for your child in showing him you cared enough to make the effort."

Meanwhile, Shirley was continuing on the journey of being Daniel's mother. Daniel seemingly was doing well enough in public school. He even won his school's spelling bee in fourth grade. But not long after that, Shirley received a disturbing phone call.

It was a mother from Daniel's school whose house was close to the bus stop: "Do you know that the other children are throwing rocks at Daniel and abusing him?" Shirley complained to the principal, who said the bus stop was out of his jurisdiction. She found out that similar things were happening at school. During recess the kids would open up his pants and pour sand in.

That was the last year Daniel would spend in that school. Shirley located a private Christian school where bullying was not tolerated. She wrote in the November 1976 newsletter about how Daniel had had trouble fitting into the public school system. Regular education hadn't been quite right, as he got distracted and could not always follow the group lessons. But special education wouldn't have been right for him either, because he had too much ability.

Shirley described the advantages of the new school's system, called Accelerated Christian Education. Children progressed at their own rate in each separate subject. Subjects were broken down into units of just three weeks; if a child failed a unit, he or she would repeat that unit only, rather than losing a whole year. A strong incentive system kept the kids progressing, and distractions were minimized by the children having their own individual study carrels instead of open desks. It was a relief to Shirley and T. G. to have Daniel in a more appropriate school.

At home, Daniel started having temper tantrums when he was around four years old. They happened when he didn't get his way over food, or other things. Over the years, Shirley worked on whittling down the tantrums. The first thing she said was, "You're not to throw things when you have a temper tantrum. I know you get angry, but you don't throw things when you're angry." Once Daniel got that under control, she started working on door slamming. She kept working her way through the misbehaviors until finally it got down to where he was just crying. Shirley told him, "That's okay. You can cry."

Another problem was that Daniel would get into the rooms of his siblings, Stephen and Ruth, and mess with their belongings. Once, he got hold of Stephen's billfold and pulled everything out, scattering the contents over the floor. Shirley solved that by putting outside-type door knobs, with keys, on

Ruth and Stephen's bedroom doors. That also gave the siblings a place to retreat to when Daniel was being insufferable.

But most of the time, the two doted on their little brother. Stephen, the oldest child, was protective from the beginning. While Shirley was still in the hospital with newborn Daniel, he overheard her on the phone with T. G. Taking the phone, Stephen said indignantly, "What do you mean, something's wrong with *our* baby?"

Some months later, after a doctor told them Daniel would be "profoundly retarded," Stephen said, "He won't stay retarded because I will teach him." Stephen figured he already knew how to do that because his teacher had assigned him to sit next to and help a boy who was developmentally delayed.

When the family went somewhere, Stephen would often carry Daniel or hold him by the hand. Ruth was also involved with him. Daniel became very attached to his brother and sister. Any time he was in a group, if there was somebody named Stephen or Ruth, Daniel automatically considered that person his best friend.

Daniel was one of six kids who attended the first-ever summer camp for PWS, run by Margo Thornley, when he was ten. Shirley spent a day at the camp and wrote about it in *The Gathered View*. For some of the kids, it was the first time they had ever been with other kids who had PWS, and they were overwhelmed. But they came to realize that they were in a place made for them. Shirley asked them what they liked about the camp:

"Nobody calls me names."
"People do things here."
"I have friends here."
"Everybody understands each other."
"Nobody picks on you."

In the safe environment Shirley created for Daniel—with his weight entirely appropriate for his height, at a school that suited him, with activities he could manage—his personality began to flower. He wanted to understand the world. Sometimes he would ask questions that would drive Shirley crazy—like, what are worms thinking about when they tunnel through the ground? He studied up on algae. He could tell you the form of glue used on stamps and envelopes (dextrin).

He also began thinking about his future. He was concerned when he found out that people with PWS were short as adults. Shirley told him, "Being five feet tall is okay." She pointed out that they had a male friend who was short, "You'll be like Mr. Donsky, he's five feet tall." Daniel seemed to accept that.

One day he asked Shirley if he'd be able to have children.

"Well, no one that's had PWS has ever had children," she said.

Daniel went to his room and shut the door. After a while he came back.

"Did that upset you when I told you that?"

"No," he said, "I'll just adopt."

As Shirley was guiding Daniel and the newsletter into their hopeful but uncertain future, Gene had an even larger responsibility. The world's first and only Prader-Willi association was in his hands. And it was turning out to be a more demanding task than he had imagined.

Six

Gene the Shepherd

G ene thought that putting out the newsletter would largely satisfy the needs of parents. He set the annual dues at five dollars, which he figured would cover expenses. But from the beginning, people wanted more: names of professionals, diet information, information on the syndrome, bibliographies, and names of nearby members. And sometimes they just wanted someone to listen.

The letters and calls to the Deterlings during the organization's first year were mainly from desperate parents who had almost given up hope. The correspondence started slowly but built up quickly. By chance, the Associated Press, *Newsweek*, and *Today's Health* articles were published during the first six months of the organization's existence. People who read the articles and called the Seattle clinic were referred to the new organization for PWS.

Gene and Fausta did their best to answer the many calls and letters, giving counsel and signing up new members. It helped tremendously that Fausta could take shorthand while stirring the soup, allowing Gene to dictate responses rapidly after coming home from work. But even so, Gene reluctantly had to pay for part-time secretarial assistance. Expenses were outstripping the dues.

Then, out of one family's tragedy, the organization received a lifeline. Susan Marie Leyshon of Silver Spring, Maryland, died from complications of PWS in August 1975, one month after the first newsletter was sent out. She was twenty-two years old. Her parents asked that expressions of sympathy take the form of contributions to Prader-Willi Syndrome Parents and Friends. The group received more than four hundred dollars—a crucial early boost.

The organization was off to a good start, growing from ten to around a hundred and fifty members in its first year. But Gene was having a hard time enjoying the success, because his business career was stalling. A couple of years before he had been flying high, as a group director with 120 people working for him. But a corporate reorganization dismantled most of his group, and Gene had the awful task of laying off 100 people.

Finally he caught a break. His boss was promoted to the corporate staff at Honeywell's headquarters in Minneapolis, and he wanted Gene to come with him. Gene would have a great job, as product director for computer peripheral equipment, overseeing worldwide activities in printers and tape drives. The only catch: the family would have to leave Harvard.

No one was happy about it but Gene. Fausta had never lived outside the Boston area. She pictured Minnesota as a great frozen forest. She was concerned about uprooting Sara and Evan, who were fifteen and thirteen at the time. But she could see how important the job was to Gene. She told herself that with Curtis so young she would be in the house with him most of the time anyway, so maybe it didn't matter so much where she lived.

Gene went to Minneapolis in spring 1976, and the rest of the family followed in summer, after the school year was over. Gene told his readers about the move in the July 1976 newsletter. He admitted that he and Fausta had been falling behind in answering the daily requests they received. But with the move behind them, he said, he would have a renewed focus on the needs of the Prader-Willi clan.

With his business career revitalized, Gene focused on building up the Prader-Willi organization. He put together a board of directors with five parents including himself, Fausta, and Shirley, and five professionals including Pipes and Holm. The board first met in Seattle on May 27, 1977, in Vanja Holm's office. For chairman, the board settled on Sam Beltran, one of the other parents, a genial and talkative anesthesiologist. The board also voted to ditch the homey "Prader-Willi Syndrome Parents and Friends" in favor of the bland but professional "Prader-Willi Syndrome Association." At least that name created a decent abbreviation: PWSA, which was lengthened to PWSA (USA) in 1992.

Gene encouraged the members to contact each other and start local groups. He wrote: "Two heads have got to be better than one, and with a dozen or so working together, the reward will probably surpass your expectations. What is really needed to get a group started is one person with initiative to contact one other person and say, 'Let's go.'" To help members find each other, he and Fausta prepared and mailed out lists of the members in each state. Shirley promoted the groups in the newsletter.

As Gene built up the organization, the newsletter continued to grow, handling difficult and important subjects. A New Jersey man, Raymond Mears, wrote to *The Gathered View* about the final days of his sixteen-year-old son with PWS. David had suffered a ruptured appendix and died three weeks after emergency surgery, from massive infection. It was a tragedy that should not have happened. Normally doctors would have detected the infected appendix and operated in time. But David rarely complained of pain throughout the ordeal, and because of that his doctors did not realize the danger he was in. His symptoms were far subtler: loss of his usual cheerfulness and aggression, and toward the end, loss of appetite.

Gene and Fausta, and Shirley and T. G. were chilled by the story. If people with PWS did not feel and report internal pain the way normal people did, then they were highly vulnerable to all sorts of internal diseases. They had thought that following Holm and Pipes's plan to keep their sons from getting obese would be enough to keep them healthy for many decades. Now they wondered if that were true.

A later article published in *The Gathered View* added to their fears. A girl from Mississippi had become listless, complaining of occasional stomach pain and losing her interest in eating. Having read the earlier article about the New Jersey boy, her mother was convinced that her daughter was seriously sick. She took her to the emergency room on a Sunday, armed with the newsletter. The doctor took the time to read the article and, because of it, admitted the girl immediately. A gallstone problem was detected and surgery performed. To the surgeon's surprise, the problem was much worse than it had seemed: the girl had chronic and acute gall bladder disease and gallstones.

At least this time there was a happy ending, as the surgery was done in time and the girl made a full recovery. Shirley and Gene could pat themselves on the back—the newsletter had made a huge difference in one girl's life. And again the doctors realized a new complication of PWS thanks to articles in the newsletter.

The organization and the newsletter were fulfilling Gene's vision of parents and professionals helping each other. In January 1977 Gene wrote, "Whereas previously so many of the letters we received had a tone of desperation and despair, we have recently noted a sign of hope and encouragement in the majority of our mail." In March 1978 he wrote, "We are now in correspondence with groups from all over the country who are enthusiastically working towards group homes, camp, and employment facilities." The organization and its newsletter had become, as one parent put it, "our bridge off of a remote island in an often cold sea."

But in some ways, raising up the organization was proving an easier task than raising up Gene and Fausta's own son. Gene's organizational savvy and optimism, and Fausta's warm and unruffled competence were meeting their match in their youngest offspring.

Seven

Quirky Curtis

C urtis was "a very cute and very round little boy with a winning smile that covers his whole face," according to his first preschool teacher, at a school for handicapped children in the Boston area. She called him "the welcoming committee for newcomers." His biggest deficit was in gross motor skills; it was hard for him to climb or pedal a tricycle. He was resistant to toilet training, and he would get annoyed if she asked him to copy something she had drawn. But overall Curtis at three to four years of age was a charmer.

His preschool teacher for the following year was not so charmed. She found that while Curtis could attend well to tasks, he was often unwilling to cooperate. He tired easily and was frequently "lazy," as she put it, about physical activities and games. He was still in diapers, at age five, and became very upset when she tried to discuss it with him.

She laid out her concerns in a year-end report: "He cannot accept corrections. Curt becomes frustrated and may lose self-confidence if he feels teacher or situation is unfair. He often fears others will get advantages he doesn't get. He does not like other children to touch or look or stare at him. And he is very selective about who he lets sit near him, if he lets anyone at all. Curtis tends to be a loner in the classroom, but he does have one friend whom he likes very much."

At home, Curtis was the same mixture of charm and prickliness. He was certainly in the mix, wanting to be with his big brother and sister and his parents. He loved picture books, cars and trucks, his family's cats, animals in general, being pushed on the swing, and watching *Sesame Street.*

And he had a mind of his own. He would get into struggles with his much older siblings and end up pointing his finger at them and shouting. Sara and Evan dubbed him "The Little King."

He had a hard time waiting for meals, or not getting something he wanted. Sometimes he would get so frustrated he would scream, or kick his feet, or throw things. He would pound the table. Other times he would badger Fausta, tugging on her and saying, "Mom, Mom, Mom, Mom. Why Mom?"

Gene remained stubbornly optimistic. Just as Curtis was finishing his second and final year of preschool, Gene issued a statement in the newsletter: "A good share of the difficulties with the syndrome relates to the lack of good dietary habits being developed in the very early formative years. With the aid of a good nutritionist and determined parents, the chances are high that the child will remain a joy rather than growing to be a burden. We have a number of letters to attest to that, and we know from experience with our own son, Curtis, that it is true. Friendly, happy, likable, fun, sensitive, thoughtful, loving—those are the characteristics of a Prader-Willi child under control."

But despite Gene's inspirational writings, it appeared that Curtis was just as prone to behavior problems as the cases of PWS described in the medical literature. As Curtis reached the age for kindergarten, in fall 1976, the Deterlings were settling in at their new home in Orono, Minnesota. Gene went to the local public elementary school, Schumann, to speak to the principal, Ron Gilbert. Gene said he wasn't sure if Curtis was ready for kindergarten. Someone on Gilbert's staff reviewed the reports on Curtis from his Massachusetts preschools and suggested to Gilbert that the school district might need to pay to place Curtis in a school for handicapped children.

But Gilbert wasn't so sure. That would be a restrictive environment, where Curtis would not have the benefit of being exposed to a mainstream classroom—and it would be expensive for the school system. He met with Curtis and told Gene afterward, "Gee, he's quite a talker. He's ready for kindergarten." But Gilbert also hedged his bet. He arranged for a school psychologist to see Curtis and do a report.

Curtis joined Doris Fenholt's kindergarten class in fall 1976. It didn't go well. He came across as very self-centered. He could not stand to take turns and wait in line. He did not learn the names of the other children and often resisted the teacher's directions about what to do next. The only thing Curtis liked about kindergarten was playing games.

Curtis was getting a reputation. Some of the older kids on the Deterlings' street decided to play a prank. They got hold of some sidewalk chalk and drew a giant wheelchair sign on the Deterlings' driveway. Curtis saw it, and he knew what it meant. Gene found out which kids had done it and called their parents.

When the psychologist met Curtis in mid-October, he was braced for a difficult time, but he found Curtis more engaging than he had expected—quirky, too. Curtis insisted on wearing his stocking cap indoors. And he tended to fixate on certain subjects. They got into a discussion of how and why flies came into the school. The psychologist explained that they came in to get warm and would die outside in the cold. Curtis continued to question and speculate about why the flies were coming in, as the psychologist tried to steer him back to test-taking.

Curtis scored close to average in verbal IQ (94) but way down at the bottom in performance IQ (53), which measures various non-verbal abilities. The psychologist attributed the low performance IQ to Curtis's lack of comprehension, tendency to get distracted, and insistence on doing things his own way rather than the way he had been told to do it. Based on the psychologist's report and the recommendation of his teacher, Gilbert proposed that Curtis transfer out of the kindergarten class for one more year of preschool. The Deterlings were fine with that. In the more relaxed setting of the Stubbs Bay Nursery and Child Development Center, Curtis did much better. His teacher saw him as friendly and talkative, with acceptable social skills, but stubborn at times.

In fall 1977 Curtis re-entered Doris Fenholt's kindergarten class. This time things went better. Fenholt was a veteran kindergarten teacher, and she had the benefit of having learned some lessons from Curtis' first, abortive year in her classroom. As the year went on she became more and more confident that she had him figured out. At the end of the year she wrote some "Hints in working with Curtis" as a guide for his future teachers.

She had learned not to go head to head with Curtis. Her advice was: "Avoid confrontation. Be sure he understands what he's to do and then leave until he is done." And she had found out how to go around his negativity and motivate him: "Curtis will say 'I can't do that' to anything new—I say, 'But I am going to teach you,' and proceed to do so. He delights in learning new things, and he will often tell you how good he is."

With an understanding teacher, Curtis did better. His case worker noted, "He often thrives on attention from his classmates now rather than the adults he leaned on so long. He does have hassles with peers and when he bugs Mrs. F about it she makes it his problem to solve. Now tears are less often and he can even take others laughing at his mistakes." Unlike the previous fall, he now knew the names of all his classmates and could stand to take turns and wait in line. Still there were some issues, as a spring progress report noted: "He continues to meddle into others' business and likes to be the 'authority' to his classmates. He still has a mind of his own and once he does it's difficult to persuade him otherwise."

As Curtis moved on to first grade, the staff at Schumann were torn between wanting him in the mainstream class as much as possible—to try to socialize and normalize him—and the fact that Curtis was very distracted by the full classroom of twenty-seven children, and could be distracting to the other children, as well. They decided to pull him out of the mainstream class for small group instruction in math, language development, and handwriting—areas in which he was well behind the class anyway—but keep him in the full class for reading and the softer subjects of social studies and science/health.

But it was difficult to keep Curtis in the mainstream class for reading. He constantly wanted reassurance that he was right or was the best—despite the fact that he was at the bottom of his class. He demanded a lot of individual attention. By January the staff had given up and switched Curtis to a small group for reading.

First grade was a letdown after Curtis's promising year in kindergarten. The kindergarten teacher had kept Curtis with the class for most of the day. But by the end of first grade, Curtis was leaving the mainstream classroom for all of his core academic instruction. The kindergarten teacher had maintained a positive attitude about Curtis, seeing him as a child who wanted to and could learn, if approached the right way. But as first grade wore on, the staff focused more and more on Curtis's liabilities.

In the middle of Curtis's discouraging first-grade experience, Gene issued another soaring statement in the newsletter. He was seeing "a much more positive tone" in his mail from parents. "The sharing experiences, the feeling of no longer being alone, and the working toward a common goal have given many a new feeling of hope. We're convinced that many of these hopes can someday be satisfied."

He acknowledged the frustration many parents were feeling (not least, himself and Fausta). But he had a stubborn faith in a better future: "To those who are still discouraged by the lack of progress they have seen in dealing with their own situation, we want to urge you not to give up hope. Some of us are more fortunate than others in having a child who responds more easily than some other Prader-Willi people to dietary measures and behavior modification. Regardless, eventually we will learn how to treat them all, and even though there will always be inequities, we can still look forward to improvement in all Prader-Willi people's futures."

The coming year, 1979, would likely see "greater progress than in all the past years put together," according to Gene. That June the world's first conferences on Prader-Willi syndrome would be held. First came a scientific conference, organized by Vanja Holm and Peggy Pipes along with Stephen Sulzbacher, their psychologist colleague. Two weeks later was a general conference put on by PWSA. It did indeed look like 1979 would be a breakthrough year.

Part II

Breakthroughs and Breakdowns

Eight

LIKE FINDING FAMILY YOU DIDN'T KNOW YOU HAD

The PWSA board, meeting in San Francisco in the summer of 1978, agreed with Gene's proposal to put on a conference in Minneapolis the following summer. At that same board meeting a second anesthesiologist, Dick Wett, joined the board of PWSA.

Dick and his wife, Marge, were Catholic and had seven children. Lisa, their daughter with PWS, was the second youngest. The cause of her problems had been a mystery until one day in October 1975 when Dick was reading his favorite magazine, *Newsweek*, and came across the description of a syndrome he had never heard of that sounded exactly like Lisa's problems. Soon he was in touch with Vanja Holm, who made the diagnosis.

Lisa was ten years old when Dick read that *Newsweek* article. Dick was philosophical about how long it took for her to be diagnosed. He told a reporter: "There are more than 3,000 syndromes. To expect every doctor to recognize PWS is not realistic."

Dick's wife, Marge, was a spark plug. Growing up in the small town of Walworth, Wisconsin, she had been a tomboy. Her brother, who was one year older than her, taught her how to drive and shoot a gun. She and her buddies would make their own slingshots, catch spiders in jars, and climb the town's water tower. They would steal melons and occasionally get shot at by farmers. Their favorite prank was to go to a nearby town, stand on their car to reach the switch that turned off the street lights, and then wait for the local sheriff to chase them.

As a mother of seven, she was more sedate—somewhat. She loved to fix up houses. While very pregnant with Lisa, her idea of fun was to haul a large roll of carpeting into a vacation cabin they had recently purchased. She would challenge her sons to arm-wrestling contests, and not until their high school years could they beat her. In the mid-1970s she took up welding because she wanted to make a metal sculpture for the front yard. Dick taught her the basics, but she wanted to learn more, so she signed up for a class at Hennepin Vo-Tech. When she showed up, the instructor said, "You're in my class?"

"Yes."

"I've never had a woman in my class before."

"Well, you do now."

The instructor showed the students a basic weld, and then left the room. All the other students started turning on their gas, trying unsuccessfully to light their torches.

"Everybody shut down, we're going to explode this place," Marge said.

The instructor still hadn't come back, so Marge showed them all how to safely light their torches, as Dick had taught her. When the instructor returned, Marge had to laugh—he hadn't had a woman in his class before, but now he had one taking over.

"Oh, well, they don't unlock the women's bathroom at this hour," the instructor said.

"Then I'll have to remember to go before I come."

Marge and Dick met the Deterlings in 1978, when Gene organized the Minnesota chapter of PWSA. At one of the early parent meetings, Gene said he could use some help running PWSA because he had to travel a lot for his job.

Marge was eager to help. She had experience, having co-founded the Edina Special Children's Group and served as its newsletter editor, secretary, and president. Marge could see that Gene was getting overwhelmed with correspondence and membership. She told Gene he had to start running things differently. He was still writing out all the names of the members in a notebook each year. Marge told him he needed to get a Rolodex, so each member's information could be written on a card and moved around so it wouldn't have to be rewritten.

Gene was resistant. He liked his notebooks. Marge tried to help him with correspondence, but again they butted heads. Finally she told him, "I want to help you but I'm sorry, I'm just battling with you all the time. You give me what you want me to do and I'll do it, but I'll do it my way." Gene capitulated. He let Marge handle membership. Then she started doing the correspondence. Bit by bit she was taking over the running of the organization.

But Gene kept control of the planning for the conference. In his mind, this was the last foundation stone he needed to put in place. If he could pull it off, then PWSA would be strong enough to stand on its own. But in the months before the conference, he began to have serious concerns. Membership growth, steady since the organization's start, stagnated.

Gene soldiered on. He lined up speakers. Vanja Holm, Hans Zellweger, Bryan Hall (who had co-written the break-through 1972 medical review about PWS in *The Journal of Pediatrics*), Margo Thornley. In the January 1979 newsletter Gene wrote that they "still had high hopes" that Andrea Prader would come from Switzerland, but in the end, Prader declined. Gene had no idea how many people might show up. Fifty? A hundred? Three hundred? He asked members to send in a non-binding form so he could get some idea, and by March 1979, more than seventy-five said they were coming. Gene settled on the Leamington Hotel in downtown Minneapolis as the venue.

One of the members planning to attend was Marilyn Bintz, a nurse from Davis, California, who had an eight-year-old daughter with PWS named Page. Marilyn traveled to Minneapolis on her own, leaving Page and her son with her husband. The night before the first day of the conference, she was too excited to sleep. She was early for breakfast, and while waiting for a table started chatting with a woman next to her, D. J. Miller, also the parent of a child with PWS.

The waitress said to them, "Table for three, this way." The waitress had assumed that a third woman standing behind them was with them. The third woman apologized for the waitress's mistake.

Marilyn said to her, "Are you here for the conference?"

"Yes."

"Then you belong with us."

The third woman's name was Gloria Means, and she and Marilyn and D. J. would be friends for many conferences to come. The whole conference went like that for Marilyn. It was like finding family that she didn't know was out there. At the end of the conference nobody wanted to go home. A group of about forty or so went out to dinner at a restaurant and stayed for hours.

One of the conference speakers made the claim that the syndrome was of Germanic origins. This struck Marilyn as dubious, as there was Gloria, who was black, sitting next to her. Marilyn also got to know Vanja Holm. At one point, everyone was talking about the short stature of people with PWS, and Holm, who was not quite five feet tall, said, "And what's bad about that?" What Marilyn took away from that conference was not any particular piece of information or wisdom, but the sense that there was this wonderful group that was going to work on the problems of PWS and not give up.

Shirley Neason was also at the first conference, and she brought Daniel. He was twelve and enjoyed being with other young people with PWS. Shirley was struck by how similarly the kids looked and behaved. She noticed how their hands would sneak into the sugar bowl and slip packets of sugar into their pockets. There were also regular temper outbursts, even in public.

Gene and Fausta were thrilled with how well the conference went. Attendance was a solid 165. It was the largest ever assembly of people concerned with Prader-Willi syndrome. Parents seemed so happy to be in a place where they could ask their questions without anyone thinking they were strange. Emotions were high. One young woman got up to ask a question and got so flustered it seemed she was about to cry. Gene stood and said, "You're doing fine, kid."

Prader may not have made it, but Hans Zellweger was there. He interviewed the children with PWS at the conference, trying to learn more about their psychology. Fausta found him warm and supportive.

Gene had prepared evaluation sheets, and many of the comments were glowing. There was strong sentiment to make the conference an annual event. Gene felt drained and relieved. He sensed that connections had been formed that would bind the organization together for many years to come. At the conference, he told the board and the members that he and Fausta planned to resign as officers in the next year. There was little doubt who would succeed them in managing the day-to-day affairs of the organization. Gene nominated Marge Wett as vice president, and the board approved.

The first PWSA conference was indeed the organizational breakthrough that Gene had hoped for. But what about his high hopes for the other conference—the first-ever scientific conference, held that same summer in Seattle? Would it lead to a breakthrough in understanding or treatment of the syndrome? Gene knew that was what the members of PWSA were hoping for above all else.

Nine

Puzzled Professionals

Sixty professionals attended the first-ever scientific conference on Prader-Willi syndrome. They had an impressive collection of initials after their names: MD, RD, BS, MS, MA, MSW, MPH, EdD, FRCP, and PhD. The biggest group was from Seattle, but attendees also came from California, Illinois, Iowa, Kansas, Minnesota, New York, and Vermont, and from British Columbia, Canada.

One of them was a young doctor from Iowa, James Hanson, who was a protégé of Hans Zellweger. Hanson's father had come of age during the Great Depression, with little money and painful malformed feet—club feet. He overcame his handicap and became a federal judge. Influenced by his father's experiences, Hanson grew fascinated with developmental disorders.

Hanson began his presentation at the conference by admitting that all the unanswered questions about PWS were frustrating for both parents and doctors. All doctors could do was treat the symptoms. Without any understanding of what caused the syndrome, there was little hope of curing or preventing it. But Hanson proposed a way forward. He noted that many of the symptoms of PWS pointed to a defect in the central nervous system, and in particular to midline structures of the brain including the hypothalamus and thalamus. Others had also noticed this, but Hanson took it a step farther: he proposed that a single defect in that brain region, early in fetal development, could be the cause of PWS.

This hypothetical brain injury might have multiple causes, environmental or genetic. This raised the possibility of prevention, at least for environmental causes. Perhaps prevention would be as simple as making sure that pregnant women avoided certain substances or got enough of other substances? Hanson urged doctors to be alert to these possibilities. Holm had already investigated the theory that a zinc deficiency might cause PWS, but she hadn't come up with good evidence for it.

Holm raised an alternative possibility in her presentation: that PWS would turn out to have a single genetic cause, like Down syndrome. Before 1959, Holm pointed out, Down syndrome had been in the same dubious category as Prader-Willi syndrome: a bunch of symptoms with no explanation for what caused them. Then, in 1956, geneticists finally figured out exactly what a normal set of human chromosomes looked like: 23 pairs of chromosomes, with one member of each pair from each parent. Once that was clear, the genetic cause of Down syndrome practically jumped out of the microscope; there was an extra copy—a third copy—of chromosome 21. But no one had seen any extra or missing chromosomes in Prader-Willi syndrome, and Holm did not believe that PWS was caused by abnormal chromosomes.

Zellweger, who knew a great deal about genetics, had looked at the evidence closely. He knew there was a hint of a genetic cause, since 8 percent of PWS cases studied had chromosome abnormalities, compared with 1 percent of the population at large. But the abnormalities were scattered among various types. Zellweger, like Holm, concluded that PWS was not caused by abnormal chromosomes.

To Gene's disappointment, there was no breakthrough on the cause of PWS at the scientific conference. Nor was there any breakthrough in management of the syndrome. Several papers proposed various types of behavior modification that seemed more appropriate for rats in a maze than human beings. For instance, Stephen Sulzbacher, Pipes and Holm's psychologist colleague, suggested that a PWS child's school lunch be divided into bite-sized portions, to be doled out for work performed: "For example, he might get a bite of his sandwich after finishing three pages in his Sullivan reader, then another bite after doing four pages of arithmetic, etc."

Zellweger proposed a set of strict rules designed to make eating a rational, utilitarian act. When young children with PWS were given what he called "feedings," the bib and table mat should always be a special bright color, used only for that occasion. Feedings should always be in the same place and at the same times, and a bell should be rung at the start of each feeding. No love or praise should be expressed during the feedings. He described his approach as Pavlovian.

The more useful presentations came from professionals who listened to what parents were telling them. Jurgen Herrmann, a social worker, was impressed by the range of problems that Prader-Willi kids presented their parents with: repetitive or incessant activities (talking, playing with puzzles, pulling hair, and picking sores), overconfidence and boasting, a manipulative personality, tiring easily and not having enough strength to keep up with peers, snitching food and other items, frequent temper tantrums, and communication difficulties because of speech delay.

Sulzbacher also was listening to parents, and he focused on a particularly difficult aspect of the syndrome: acting out and noncompliance. Parents had told him that their children's anxiety levels seemed to rise before temper tantrums, so he was experimenting with ways to reduce their anxiety and hopefully make them more cooperative. These included biofeedback, meditation and tai chi.

Perhaps the most helpful presentation came from Peggy Pipes, who repeated her common-sense advice on strict control of the food environment. Her new discovery was how critical it was to start young: "If the diagnosis is made in early childhood, the child, family, and everybody in the environment learns to accept the fact that the child has a disorder that needs special treatment (a low calorie diet). The earlier in the child's life that this understanding occurs, the more likely it seems that the result will be a rational approach to a difficult problem."

But it was a hard syndrome to diagnose early. Many doctors would recognize it only once the child had become obese—and often missed the diagnosis even then. If only the cause of PWS were known. Then there could be a lab test, a definitive way to diagnose it at a very young age. Then families would know what they were facing and would have a better chance to cope and grow with the syndrome. But the North American professionals at the Seattle conference could only speculate on the cause of PWS.

Across the Atlantic, however, a different set of researchers—completely unknown to Gene—had something better than speculation: a clue.

Ten

The Europeans Sniff Out A Clue

For Christopher Hawkey, 1974 was a very good year. Hawkey was a lanky twenty-seven-year-old English doctor with an intense but kindly air. He was still a trainee, doing a rotation in endocrinology and nutrition at Northwick Park Hospital in the Greater London Area. He'd taken the job at Northwick not primarily for the work, but because the program offered married quarters. It was the first time he and his wife were able to live together under the same roof, and that's why 1974 was such a good year. Their first child was born the following year.

Hawkey was working at a clinical research center focused on obesity when he met Cedric, a new patient. Hawkey's role was to do the initial exam and get a history. At first glance, Cedric seemed like just another obesity patient, albeit quite short at five feet one inch tall. Then Hawkey noticed that Cedric, an adult, was reading a *Janet and John* book, for children. "Hang on," Hawkey thought to himself. Looking closely at Cedric, it just seemed like he had some kind of a syndrome.

Cedric had all the symptoms of Prader-Willi syndrome, but Hawkey did not make the diagnosis. He couldn't—he had never heard of PWS. The diagnosis was made by the clinic's endocrinologist, Richard Himsworth, who told Hawkey to write a case study on Cedric. It would be a good opportunity for the young doctor to publish something. Prader-Willi syndrome was still a relatively rare and novel thing. Himsworth also suggested that Hawkey work with Alison Smithies, the geneticist at Northwick Park who could analyze Cedric's chromosomes for any abnormalities.

Hawkey embraced the assignment, spending hours reading every medical journal article he could find on Prader-Willi syndrome. He was fascinated by the odd combination of symptoms and the mystery surrounding what the *British Medical Journal* had called, a few years before, this "obscure [but] interesting syndrome."

Then it got even more interesting. Smithies took Hawkey into her lab and showed him how she used special dyes on Cedric's chromosomes, producing distinctive light and dark bands that allowed her to identify the number of every chromosome. Before this technique, it had been hard to tell similar-sized chromosomes apart, and geneticists had often lumped chromosomes into groups—such as the D group, for chromosomes 13, 14, and 15.

The result: Cedric had a highly unusual abnormality. Normally each chromosome is separate from every other one, but Cedric's two chromosome 15s had fused together. This was the result of a "translocation"—an event in which chromosomes, or parts of them, ended up jumbled—like putting together a Lego set and getting a piece stuck in the wrong place. Sometimes translocations cause no problems. Many entirely normal people have translocations in their chromosomes. But at other times, some of the genetic material gets lost, or "deleted."

Could Cedric's Prader-Willi syndrome have been caused by a deletion of one or more genes on one or both of his chromosome 15s? It was hard to say. Hawkey could only find only one other published case of a person whose two chromosome 15s had fused, but this person did not have Prader-Willi syndrome. And there was the fact that the vast majority of people with PWS had normal-looking chromosomes. However, there were a handful of previous reports of abnormalities of D group chromosomes in Prader-Willi syndrome. Since the D group included chromosome 15, perhaps those earlier cases had also involved chromosome 15?

Hawkey and Smithies ended their paper, which was published in 1976, by calling for researchers to re-analyze cases of PWS with abnormal chromosomes using the latest techniques. There was a quick response from other European researchers. Within a year three other cases of Prader-Willi syndrome with a 15-15 translocation were reported, by teams in Italy, Switzerland and France. And two similar cases were found in 1978 and 1979, the first by the same Italian and Swiss researchers, the second by a Czech team.

The French team pointed out that such cases were unlikely to happen by chance. PWS was rare enough, and 15-15 translocations were very rare. Surely there was some causal connection between chromosome 15 and Prader-Willi syndrome? The Swiss and Italian researchers agreed. There was "little doubt," they wrote, "that chromosome 15 is involved in the pathogenesis of this syndrome."

But the North American researchers gathered for the 1979 Seattle conference were not impressed. Sure, there was a sprinkling of Prader-Willi cases in patients with defects of chromosome 15, but scores of other Prader-Willi patients had chromosomes that looked normal. They were unconvinced that chromosome 15 defects caused Prader-Willi syndrome. But they were about to face something that would be impossible to ignore.

Eleven

A Missing Piece

"Stupid endocrinologist. Everyone knows Prader-Willi syndrome is not a chromosome disorder."

Vic Riccardi was an MD with a specialty in genetics, and he ran the Kleberg Cytogenetics Laboratory at Baylor College of Medicine in Houston. He was reacting to a new order from some pediatric endocrinologist on the Baylor faculty who wanted a chromosome analysis of a girl with PWS. Waste of time, Riccardi thought. One of his top technicians, a grad student named David Ledbetter, overheard him. Ledbetter had come across Hawkey and Smithies's paper three years earlier, right after it was published. Ledbetter wasn't sure Riccardi was right, and he told him so.

Riccardi had grown up without much money in Southern California. His father had a boat launching hoist in Long Beach. Riccardi used to do boat repairs underwater, without any gear, holding his breath. He was the first in his family to graduate high school. He went on to UCLA and Georgetown University School of Medicine.

He'd almost died on July 23, 1972—coincidentally, in the town of Harvard, Massachusetts, just months after the Deterlings moved there. Riccardi had been showing off for his wife, doing a running dive into a shallow pond. He had done this dive before, but this time the water level was lower. Some kids had kicked stones out of the dam the night before. His head caught on the sand, and his neck broke. He came to a stop face down in the water. He could see his wife's feet nearby but couldn't move. She watched him for a while, thinking he was showing her how long he could hold his breath.

After a minute, she reached down and turned him over, saving him from drowning. He spent weeks in the hospital. He recovered, but with permanent damage on his right side. He walked awkwardly and his hand was gnarled. But his ambition was intact. He went on to become a professor and start a number of genetics clinics.

Ledbetter was tall, with a goatee and a commanding bass voice. He fell in love with chromosomes the first time he peered at them through a microscope. They were beautiful and complex, and he could stare at them for hours. His PhD research was on monkey evolution and genetics. He had taken the job at Riccardi's lab to make money, but he was increasingly intrigued by human genetics.

A few days later it was time for the weekly sign-out conference, when the whole staff sat around a large table while Riccardi led the discussion of the week's cases. When he got to the girl with PWS, he announced "Oh, David and I have a bet on this case. He thinks chromosome 15 translocations might cause Prader-Willi syndrome because there was a paper from England suggesting this a couple of years ago, and I told him I thought that was a bunch of junk. Let's see who's right."

He reviewed the results: "Normal female chromosomes. No translocation of chromosome 15—I win."

Riccardi closed the folder and passed it around the table so the techs could take a look for themselves, and moved on to the next case. When the folder got to Ledbetter, he opened it and took a close look at the photos of the girl's two chromosome 15s. True, there was no translocation, but there was something else, something much subtler. One of the two 15s looked a little shorter than the other, and it also looked paler in a region of the chromosome called "proximal 15q." This suggested that there might be a small piece missing.

After staring at the photos for a few minutes, Ledbetter interrupted Riccardi: "I think the two 15s in this girl are discrepant—one looks shorter than the other, and there may be a deletion."

Riccardi wasn't having it. "David, give up. You lost the bet already. There's no translocation, so now you're trying to make up a deletion."

After the meeting, Ledbetter went back to the lab to look at the slides of the girl's chromosomes under the microscope. Now it looked even clearer to him. He got Susie Airhart, the lead technician, to come and look. She agreed that one of the girl's 15s looked "fishy."

She encouraged him to convince Riccardi to pursue the lead. Ledbetter spent a couple of hours scanning and taking pictures, then went to Riccardi's office. This time, Riccardi didn't dismiss him. Airhart and Ledbetter both had a talent for cytogenetics, and if they both thought this was worth pursuing, then Riccardi was going to pay attention. But Riccardi also knew that proximal 15q was a troublesome region. Often there was a scrunching of the light and dark bands that could mislead you into thinking there was a deletion. So Riccardi decided to set up a "blind" test, to see if Ledbetter could really distinguish the Prader-Willi girl's chromosomes from other chromosomes when he didn't know what he was looking at. He contacted the endocrinologist who had submitted the sample and got permission to talk to the girl's family. He found out the girl's name was Caroline. Riccardi persuaded Caroline's parents to give him blood samples. He also mixed in samples from a normal, unrelated female.

A month or two later the samples arrived, and Riccardi worked with one of the other technicians to do a high-resolution study. This was a new technique, and Riccardi's lab was one of the few in the country that could do it. The result: Ledbetter could easily see which of the three female samples was Caroline's. Airhart could also see it—with the high-resolution banding, she could actually see two missing bands, a light one and a dark one. Riccardi was somewhat impressed but immediately pointed out this was only one case.

Other people in the lab were dubious about the supposed deletion. The fuzzy technology—staring at blurry photos—did not make it easy. It was a judgment call, and many wondered about Ledbetter's judgment. Their attitude was, "David, you're crazy. It's just normal variation." Riccardi also doubted Ledbetter's judgment. He told Airhart that Ledbetter had a bee in his bonnet about this chromosome 15 thing and wouldn't let go of it.

Airhart found herself in the middle. She was a favorite of Riccardi's. He had made her his head technician. She was also close to Ledbetter (they would later marry). She could sense Ledbetter's passion to make a scientific discovery. It also seemed like partly a "guy testosterone thing," as she put it, a competition between Riccardi and Ledbetter about who was right. But Ledbetter also needed Riccardi. As head of the lab, Riccardi could make things happen. Ledbetter had to appeal to Riccardi's scientific curiosity. He needed reinforcements, and he got them from Europe. He dug out the other translocation cases showing abnormalities in proximal 15q in cases of PWS—the cases from Switzerland, Italy, France, and Czechoslovakia. He went into Riccardi's office and showed him. It's not just Caroline, Ledbetter told him.

Now Riccardi was intrigued. He quickly thought up a harder test. He called Jack Crawford, the head of genetics at Massachusetts General Hospital, whom he knew from his fellowship there. He said, "Jack, I'm sitting here in my office with Dave Ledbetter, graduate student, technician. If you'll send me some patient samples with PWS mixed in with normal controls, we'll tell you which is PWS and which is not."

A few months later, ten samples arrived from Massachusetts General, identified only by number. They were set up for high-resolution analysis, and Ledbetter and Airhart went to work.

They agreed that four of the samples had a proximal 15q deletion, while the other six looked normal. Ledbetter waited anxiously as Riccardi called Crawford to break the code. The result: they had nearly nailed it, identifying deletions in three of the four patients with PWS. But there were two discrepancies: Ledbetter and Airhart had identified a deletion in one of the normal samples, and they had failed to see a deletion in one of the Prader-Willi samples.

Rich Strobel, another technician, figured out what had gone wrong with the first discrepancy. That sample came from a person with a normal variation that fooled them into thinking there was a deletion. Once that was understood, it was clear that the person did not have a deletion.

But the lab could find no reason for the second discrepancy—the person with Prader-Willi syndrome who did not seem to have a deletion. They looked at a number of the patient's cells, hoping to find at least some that had the deletion. But they all looked normal. They scrutinized the description of the patient's symptoms, wondering if he might have been misdiagnosed. But he had all the symptoms of PWS.

Despite the one patient they could not explain, it was an undeniable breakthrough. Combining these results with Caroline's, the lab had now seen a proximal 15q deletion in four out of five patients with PWS, and had not seen the deletion in any of the normal controls. They had identified a previously unknown and highly specific genetic error in 80 percent of the cases of PWS they had looked at. This was a career-making discovery. Now Riccardi was fully on board—delighted, in fact. It was another coup for his lab. Just the previous year, they had co-discovered a microdeletion syndrome on chromosome 11 with another lab.

Ledbetter, Airhart, and Riccardi began working on a manuscript to submit to the prestigious *New England Journal of Medicine*. They also submitted an abstract of their work in late June 1980 for the annual meeting of the American Society of Human Genetics, to be held that September in New York City. Two months later, Riccardi told Ledbetter the good news: not only had their abstract been accepted for the meeting, it had been selected for the plenary session. This meant it had been designated as one of the top ten submissions and would be presented in a large hall to all two thousand attendees.

Now the whole Baylor genetics department got involved in honing the presentation. Riccardi was impressed with how well Ledbetter accepted all the suggestions. Often junior scientists had trouble cutting down their presentations to a manageable length, but not Ledbetter.

One question needed answering: should Ledbetter or Riccardi be the one to make the presentation at the plenary session? Riccardi told Ledbetter that someone at the American Society of Human Genetics had suggested it should be the senior researcher. But Ledbetter felt it was his discovery, and he deserved the brass ring. Riccardi acceded.

At the genetics society meeting, Ledbetter took the podium and addressed the giant hall. His presentation stirred up a lot of discussion and excitement. Prader-Willi syndrome was no longer obscure among geneticists—and neither was Ledbetter.

More than once, he was referred to as "Dr. Ledbetter." It was hard to remember that he was still a graduate student. The article came out in the February 5, 1981 issue of the *New England Journal of Medicine*. Less than a month later, Ledbetter received his PhD.

And then Ledbetter took Riccardi's place. It was an open secret at the lab that Riccardi was not on good terms with the chairman of the Baylor genetics department. Riccardi was eased out of the directorship of the lab around the time of the New York City genetics meeting. Airhart, Ledbetter and Strobel had been informally running the lab since then, under the nominal guidance of a faculty member. But shortly after Ledbetter got his PhD, he was named the new director of the Kleberg Cytogenetics Laboratory.

Holm, Pipes, and Sulzbacher were just finishing compiling papers from the 1979 scientific conference into a book when they first heard about the microdeletions. They were excited; finally, there seemed to be a clear genetic explanation for PWS. But they were also cautious, wondering about that one patient who did not have the deletion.

Ledbetter and Riccardi speculated that the one patient without a visible deletion had a smaller deletion in the same region, one beyond their ability to detect. They figured that as techniques improved they would be able to see smaller and smaller defects in proximal 15q, and eventually all patients with PWS would turn out to have a deletion in that region.

As Gene had hoped, 1979 was indeed a breakthrough year for PWS—but not, as he'd thought, because of the scientific conference in Seattle. Rather, 1979 was a breakthrough year because that was when David Ledbetter, at a lab in Houston, first stared at the chromosomes of a girl with PWS and noticed that something was missing.

Prader-Willi syndrome was going through a transition. It was no longer a mere collection of symptoms. Now it was associated with a specific microdeletion on chromosome 15. Now it had the attention of geneticists; it was nearly a proper syndrome. PWSA was also going through a transition. Gene and Fausta and Shirley had succeeded in raising it up to be a proper organization. But the organization had grown beyond their ability to manage it.

Twelve

Marge Rising

Marge Wett continued to take over PWSA. In addition to being named vice president at the June 1979 conference, she was chosen as the first chair of fund-raising. At the start of 1980, Gene agreed to transfer all secretarial duties from Fausta to Marge. He also announced that PWSA's address would henceforth be the Wetts' house. For the first time since the founding of the organization five years earlier, the Deterlings' house was no longer the headquarters.

As Marge gathered more and more of PWSA into her arms, Gene was inching toward the exit. He kept trying to build up the organization, urging members to support the founding of group homes for people with PWS and to volunteer for seven new committees the board had created to deal with specific issues. In the May 1980 newsletter he wrote, "I am not terribly happy to announce this, but on July 1st I will be resigning from my position as president of the Association." He sounded like a man still convincing himself he had to go: "When my wife and I, along with Shirley Neason, founded the organization in early 1975, we did not fully realize the effort that would be involved. The fact of the matter is that I am unable to spend the time that is required."

By the next newsletter, his last as president, he was able to write a peaceful good-bye. He celebrated the thirty-four people with Prader-Willi syndrome who came to the second conference that summer on Cape Cod: "They each brought their own distinct personalities, their own private concerns, and their own physical and mental capabilities. They displayed the same variety of humanness that the rest of us have. It was only the range of capability that was limited. But they carried their burden with a smile and friendly warmth that should make any parent as proud of them as of any child."

He was proud that the organization had been established, and proud of the support of the members. He thought PWSA would be "perpetuated forever...barring any tragic and unanticipated events." It had been an overwhelming amount of work, he admitted, but it had all been worthwhile.

It took two people to replace Gene. A new position was created for Marge: executive director. She would handle the day-to-day operations of PWSA. The new president was Sam Beltran, formerly chairman of the board. With Gene on his way out, Shirley also found herself eyeing the exit. There had always been some communications problems, with Gene in Minneapolis and Shirley in Seattle. Items had to be mailed back and forth, and long-distance phone calls were expensive. There were occasional misunderstandings. Sometimes Gene would have liked to see more of the newsletter before it was printed. It struck Shirley that with the headquarters firmly established in Marge's household, it just made sense for Marge to find someone in Minneapolis to edit the newsletter. Gene agreed, and so did Marge.

Shirley wrote her own farewell one issue before Gene's. Editing the newsletter had been exciting and rewarding, she wrote. And even more thrilling were the telephone calls, sometimes late at night or very early in the morning, from desperate people. Shirley felt she had been fulfilling a worthy purpose. She thanked the members for their letters of encouragement and support, for sending in stories, and for caring about people with PWS.

But although Shirley and Gene would no longer be actively running the association, they planned to stay involved. Gene decided that after resigning as president he would take the new position of secretary-treasurer. He and Fausta would also remain on the board.

Shirley was eager for the next phase. She would be able to write more, now that she was no longer editing the newsletter. She already had a growing list of writing credits. Besides the handbook for parents—PWSA's premiere publication, which was advertised on the back of each newsletter—she had also written an article about PWS for *Home Life*, a Baptist publication that was nationally distributed, and an article on PWS in adults that was published at the first PWSA conference.

And she discovered she could do more than write and edit. She had traveled to Vancouver to give a speech to parents; she remembered all the little sighs of relief around the room as she described the typical PWS behavioral problems and parents realized that it wasn't all their fault. She helped found the PW Association Northwest and was the group's secretary. She came up with the idea of creating national committees within PWSA to focus on areas of need, like group homes, research, and clinic services. And the board chose her to be the new vice president of PWSA.

Moreover, Shirley was the mother of arguably the most successful child with Prader-Willi syndrome to come out of Holm and Pipes's Seattle clinic. Readers of *The Gathered View* knew that Daniel was slim. He had won a spelling bee. He could jog with his father. He was in a classroom with normal kids. These were achievements that would have amazed the doctors of the 1960s.

Gene and Fausta also had projects they continued to work on. There was the local Minnesota Prader-Willi group that Gene started, and there was the project to open a Prader-Willi group home in the Minneapolis area.

Perhaps the best reward for Gene and Fausta and Shirley after their half decade of hard work was that they now could focus more fully on their youngest children. Curtis was having his challenges in school, and Daniel was entering his teen years. Both kids would need all the attention their parents could provide.

Thirteen

DANIEL AND SHIRLEY MOVE ON

Gene announced in the November 1978 newsletter that PWSA was failing to take into account the views of people with Prader-Willi syndrome. He urged them to write in so their parents and caregivers could learn how people with PWS "think, fear, love, hate, work, worry, and aspire." Shirley prodded Daniel to write something. His letter was published in the May 1979 newsletter, when he was twelve:

> "Dear Gathered View: My name is Daniel Neason. Do you know what I do? I act like a Prader-Willi. I eat food that I'm not supposed to have. Why can't I eat it? Because my weight goes up! Then what do I do? I cut down on my food situation. What happens then? My weight goes down a little bit at a time. Now what do you think will happen? I will get higher privileges on

my food situation. My problems are that when I get married my wife cannot or might not produce babies. I would have to adopt babies or marry a widow with children or babies. I cannot have food with sugar in it. I can only eat a certain amount."

Daniel did not consider himself handicapped; whatever his problems were, he would find a way around them. He saw kids with cerebral palsy, or Down syndrome, when he went to the monthly Prader-Willi clinic at the University of Washington, and that was what he considered handicapped—not him.

He had an idea about the work he wanted to do as an adult. He and Russell Iverson—Peggy Pipes's first Prader-Willi patient—were planning to open a diet gourmet restaurant. Russell's mother was pretty sure that was a bad idea—the business would last only as long as it took Russell and Daniel to consume the inventory.

Shirley was also amused by the restaurant scheme. That wasn't the answer, but she did expect Daniel to work and be independent when he grew up. At the same time, she knew he would need support. There were definite gaps in his abilities. He could memorize math facts but couldn't apply them. If you told him he had 100 apples and 10 bags, and he needed to put an equal number of apples in each bag, he wouldn't know whether to add, subtract, multiply, or divide.

Daniel's school closed just as he finished sixth grade. Shirley was able to find another one that followed the same Christian curriculum. Daniel started seventh grade there in fall 1979.

His new teacher noticed that Daniel had trouble with the "th" sound and would say, "fank you very much." Shirley had never focused on it as it seemed the least of his problems. But his teacher worked on it and got him to pronounce "th" correctly. Daniel's eyes were opened. He told his mom, "I always thought I heard people saying F."

It was a good school and a good year. But Daniel still struggled at times with his temper. Shirley's hard work in limiting his tantrums did not always carry over to the school setting. In spring 1980, he started screaming and cursing after his teacher reprimanded him. Then he felt remorseful and started to cry, saying "I don't think I'll go to heaven." The teacher was a missionary on furlough. He took Daniel into his office and told him it's Jesus who forgives your sins and takes you to heaven; it's not what you do.

Thanks to Shirley's oversight, Daniel was trim. Nonetheless, he developed scoliosis, and his orthopedist gave him a body cast to wear. Daniel didn't like wearing the cast, but he put up with it. On Sunday, June 1, Daniel and his parents were having their noon meal. Daniel had had a cold for a couple of weeks and was feeling lousy. He complained about the cast: "Oh Daddy, it hurts—take it off!"

T. G. took off the cast. Daniel was listless for the rest of the day, but he did go with Shirley and T. G. to church that evening. During the service he said he didn't feel well and wanted to sit in the car. Shirley stayed afterward for choir practice, and T. G. drove Daniel home.

When Shirley got home, T. G. told her Daniel had been vomiting. That was unusual. People with PWS rarely vomit.

Shirley wasn't sure what to make of it. Other people were suffering from some bug that was making them vomit—sometimes as they were crawling to the bathroom—or pass out. Daniel probably had the same thing.

The next day she took him to the doctor. "Oh, this is going around," the doctor told her. He gave Daniel suppositories to try to relieve the vomiting. That Monday and the next day Daniel did not eat anything and just sat around the house. He vomited more on Tuesday and occasionally passed out. Shirley called the doctor, who said to keep giving him the suppositories. If Daniel was not better the next day, the doctor said he would hospitalize him.

That evening Daniel said he was feeling better, although he had huge dark circles under his eyes. Shirley considered staying up with him but decided she needed to get her rest, since if he were hospitalized the next day, she would be staying with him in the hospital. She and T. G. kissed him good night and tucked him into bed. They told him to call them if he needed anything in the night. Shirley left Daniel's bedroom door open and hers, as well, and kept the lights on.

The next morning Shirley woke and went looking for Daniel, but he wasn't in his bed. She went to his bathroom. She found him on the floor, motionless. He had passed away from this world.

That same day the last newsletter that Shirley had edited came to her in the mail—she always mailed one to herself. Later it seemed to her she had been touched by prophecy when she had told Gene months earlier that he should find another editor.

The shock gave way to grief, but Shirley had things to do. That same evening she called Fausta, who felt terrible; the news was crushingly sad. After hanging up, Fausta started to worry. How could Daniel have died in the bathroom like that? Had he ingested something? That was the thing—what had he ingested?

Shirley and T. G. wanted to know what had happened, too. They asked for an autopsy. When the death certificate arrived, it gave the cause as myocarditis—inflammation of heart muscle. Shirley enlisted Vanja Holm's help in understanding what had happened. Holm was also devastated by the news. After consulting with pediatric cardiologists, Holm's opinion was that the virus had invaded Daniel's heart, causing it to swell and go into fibrillation.

The second PWSA conference was just two weeks after Daniel's death. Shirley composed herself and made the trip to Cape Cod. As planned, she was named vice president. Everyone wanted her to stay involved, and so did Shirley. She was active at the board meeting, arguing successfully to create a new committee on education. She also wrote a letter for the newsletter. She thanked the readers for the cards and letters of sympathy. They were especially welcome because they kept trickling in long after the initial flood from friends and relatives had dried up.

She continued, "I know many parents are concerned because they are aware that Daniel's weight had been under control since early childhood, and all had hoped that weight control would result in longer life for our children." But she reassured the readers that his death was "in no way directly related to Prader-Willi syndrome." A common, everyday virus, in a rare fluke, had made its way to Daniel's heart. She wished all of the readers "many more precious years with the Prader-Willi person in your life" and vowed to stay active in PWSA, because in her heart she would always be a "Prader-Willi parent."

Shirley had chosen her words carefully. She wrote that Daniel's death was not "directly related" to his having PWS. But privately she wondered if, like the boy with appendicitis and the girl with gallbladder disease, Daniel also failed to feel the pain that a normal person would have felt. Maybe Prader-Willi syndrome had covered up the severity of what was happening inside him. She wondered if she should have been more aggressive with the doctor.

But in the end she accepted that God had His reasons for taking Daniel. She thought maybe she could understand the timing, as Daniel was facing the most difficult part of his life— the teen years and the inevitable growing gap between himself and his peers, between his aspirations and his limitations.

She also felt grateful to the teacher at the Baptist school who had reassured Daniel that his misbehavior would not keep him from Heaven, that Jesus forgave sins. She was glad Daniel knew that before he died.

After Daniel's death, the Neasons started having a problem with the toilet in his bathroom. When T. G. investigated, he found several packages of food stashed in the toilet tank. It was Daniel's final covert op.

Shirley had every intention of staying active with PWS, but it didn't work out. The social workers at the monthly PWS clinic at the University of Washington asked her to stop coming. They told Shirley that the new parents were discouraged by the presence of someone who had lost a child. Without the monthly trips to the university, Shirley wasn't getting any new information.

And so Shirley Neason, co-founder and vice president of PWSA, first editor of *The Gathered View*, and author of the handbook for parents, slipped away from the world of PWS. She found a different outlet for her nurturing talents, becoming a kindergarten teacher at another private Christian school. When the papers from the first PWS scientific conference were published in 1981, Peggy Pipes and Vanja Holm wrote: "This book is dedicated to the memory of Daniel Neason (1966–1980), one of our earliest patients, for whom we had high hopes."

It was a lonelier world for Gene and Fausta after Daniel's death. The trail they were on looked more forbidding without Shirley scouting ahead. Meanwhile, Curtis's problems were mounting.

Fourteen

CURTIS VERSUS ELEMENTARY SCHOOL

In the fall of second grade, the staff at Schumann Elementary had a conference with Gene and Fausta. The staff concluded that Curtis was stubborn, noncompliant, and manipulative at home as well as school. Time-outs were used to try to calm and redirect him.

The problems increased in third grade. Curtis was talking back to the Schumann staff and sometimes striking out physically. The staff responded by clamping down. Ron Gilbert, the principal, took over discipline. This worked for a while, but eventually Gilbert lost his taste for dealing directly with Curtis.

By the end of third grade, the Schumann staff realized they needed help. They referred Curtis's case to District 287, a consortium of twelve Minneapolis-area school districts that dealt with issues beyond the capabilities of a single district. An evaluation was scheduled for late fall.

The staff also added more support for dealing with Curtis. He was assigned to a male teacher, Mr. Cooper, for fourth grade. The staff was also able to procure a management aide who would be assigned exclusively to Curtis. Mrs. Corcoran was hired to fulfill that role. In October Gilbert asked her to write a daily log, to document Curtis's behavior problems for the District 287 people.

Corcoran's first log entry was dated October 13, 1981. Curtis was incorrectly using the playground swing. He was told to obey the rules, but he refused. Cooper came out and told Curtis to stay behind on the playground when the rest of the class entered the building. Curtis tried to go inside with his class, but Cooper detained him. Curtis argued. Cooper told him to be quiet.

Once Curtis quieted down, Cooper reminded him that he was required to follow the rules of the playground, then told him he was free to rejoin the class. But instead of going in quietly, Curtis called Cooper a nincompoop. Cooper grabbed Curtis and shook him, saying he did not expect Curtis to call him a name since he had never called Curtis one. Curtis spent the next twenty minutes standing by a locker, crying and picking at a fleck of paint. Eventually he calmed down and joined his class for physical education.

And so it went that fall. There were daily battles of will between Curtis and the staff, sometimes escalating to the physical. Sometimes they involved food. On one occasion some egg fell on the floor of the lunchroom and Curtis ate it before Corcoran could grab it. He also tried to eat the rind of his melon. "Melon a disaster," wrote Corcoran.

Three weeks later Curtis was having a hard day. "Ornery," wrote Corcoran. He wasn't accepting any suggestions from his teachers. His mantra was "I'll do it myself!" He got frustrated at lunch because Fausta had packed the wrong juice. After lunch he flew into a rage when Corcoran insisted he do schoolwork instead of a fun page of puzzles. Corcoran and Ms. Clark, a special education teacher, carried him, thrashing, out of the room. On the way out he banged his arm on the door. He stayed just outside the door the rest of the period, crying.

He didn't show up the next day. Fausta called to find out what had happened, as Curtis was favoring his arm. Corcoran told her it was most likely the result of his thrashing about the previous day. The following day, Curtis was back. He was cheerful and worked nicely all day. Sometimes there were good days.

Not long after the previous incident, Corcoran introduced him to the concept of money, and of one cent also being $.01. Curtis argued against the idea, insisting that one cent was the same as one dollar. He became obnoxious, and Corcoran left him alone. Curtis continued to mumble: "You should be fired and sent back to school. You are too stupid to know what I know."

The next day things got worse. Curtis told Corcoran that she was not allowed to go with him on an upcoming field trip. She was annoyed by his bossy attitude. She told him to be respectful, and that if he didn't do what he was supposed to do she would call Fausta and he would have to go home.

Curtis then practiced passive resistance, refusing to leave the room when he was supposed to. After waiting several minutes, Corcoran came up with a plan to get him to move. She grabbed his favorite pencil box from his desk and left the room. Curtis was outraged. He ran out of the room and smacked Corcoran in the back.

Curtis was sent home with a disciplinary referral for having struck Corcoran. The sheet also stated that Curtis had shown regret: "Curtis has apologized to Mrs. Corcoran. Further incidents will result in temporary suspension." But Corcoran had reason to doubt the sincerity of Curtis's apology, as he told her the next day that it was not bad to hit teachers.

Finally the day arrived for the representatives from District 287 to observe Curtis. Jeanne Johnson, a school psychologist, came along with another staffer. They observed Curtis during a music class with his peers, and Johnson did some math with Curtis. Corcoran was amazed—and not entirely pleased—to see how well Curtis behaved himself around the District 287 observers. He did not throw a single fit. He was not even a little bit sassy.

Corcoran felt like Curtis was putting on an act. She wanted the District 287 observers to see the Curtis she knew. She showed them her log. But she wanted them to get a live performance, as well, so she tried to trigger a tantrum.

She had an opportunity after the music rehearsal while Curtis was holding onto a Speak and Spell game. She told him to put it down. He resisted. She grabbed it from his hands. He tried to push the buttons on it, but Corcoran blocked him, placing herself between Curtis and the game. Curtis did not take the bait. He sat down and mildly told Corcoran she was not his boss. The next day Corcoran felt bad for having tried to trigger a tantrum. She decided she would be very nice to Curtis the whole day and avoid all confrontations.

Johnson wrote her report ten days later. She had been expecting an obese child, based on what she had read about Prader-Willi syndrome, but Curtis looked only slightly chubby or stout. She found him to be fairly verbal. He was cooperative and socially appropriate with her, and she observed him being appropriate with peers on two or three occasions.

She acknowledged the problems documented in Corcoran's log and Clark's estimate that Curtis had four or five temper tantrums a day at school. But she didn't think the problems should be blamed only on Prader-Willi characteristics, which she described as a lack of emotional control and "sporadic negativism." She called out the staff—Corcoran in particular—for engaging in continuous power struggles with Curtis. She saw Curtis as an insecure and anxious kid who was using passive-aggressive techniques to try to get some control over his environment. She admonished the school for providing little, if any, positive reinforcement.

Johnson urged school staff to think creatively. They needed a behavior management plan with a strong emphasis on positive reinforcement. She also hoped Curtis could get more time with his peers—she thought he was too isolated from them because of Corcoran's presence and because he spent so much time in the special education resource room.

The Schumann staff tried to meet Johnson's challenge. They developed a behavior modification program. Curtis would earn stickers and stars for specific behaviors: not arguing with an adult for more than five minutes out of each half hour, getting to class on time in the morning and after recess, taking off his boots, and washing his hands (he didn't like to wash his hands after using the toilet).

He could redeem the stickers and stars for thirty minutes of fun time in the afternoon and an occasional popcorn party. There were also negative consequences: time-outs or going to Gilbert's office. Arguing for half an hour with an adult would result in the loss of a star. Fausta signed off on the plan.

Curtis was happy with the rewards he could earn under the new program. For the first few days, the program worked well, motivating Curtis to limit his arguing and do what he was supposed to do. At times the program was itself a distraction—Curtis would argue about whether he had been arguing. Overall, though, it was a good start.

But one week after the program was implemented, Curtis and Corcoran had their worst blowup yet. It started at morning recess, when Curtis did not follow rules and was loud and sassy. Corcoran warned him he would have to go to Clark's room for a time-out if he didn't quiet down. Curtis started shouting. Corcoran and another teacher dragged a thrashing Curtis to Clark's room. Corcoran and Cooper decided to take away the popcorn party he had earned. Curtis was in a rage, shaking his fist at Corcoran.

Eventually he quieted down, and they let him out. Lunch went okay. After lunch Curtis refused to let Corcoran help him with subtraction, shouting that she was too stupid to know how to subtract. She took away a puzzle that was distracting him. He came at her, swinging with two hands and kicking. She blocked him, but he was able to land one blow. Corcoran hit him across the face. Curtis stopped attacking and yelled "Teachers shouldn't hit children!" Cooper and another male teacher forced Curtis into his seat. Half an hour later Curtis had not regained control. The staff decided to send him home.

They called Fausta, who came to the school. Curtis told her he didn't want to go home. Corcoran offered to have Cooper and the other male teacher drag Curtis to Fausta's car, but Fausta did not want to do it that way. She requested that Curtis be put in time-out in an empty room, so he could regain control. Corcoran and the other staff were frustrated with Fausta, feeling she was not supporting their attempts to discipline Curtis, and Fausta was frustrated with the school staff for continuing their power struggles with Curtis.

Finally Curtis broke the logjam by deciding to go home with Fausta. There was a cooling-off period, as Curtis went to Arizona with his parents the next day. When Curtis returned to school nearly a week later, both he and the staff were able to reset. Corcoran told him that from now on, any adult at the school could give him a pink slip for misbehavior. She reviewed all the rules with him, and reminded him that he would have to pay for pink slips by missing part of recess. The clearly defined positive and negative consequences did help Curtis to be better behaved for the remainder of the school year. He had more good days and fewer bad days. He earned a number of fun afternoon times and popcorn parties, along with a pile of pink slips.

Despite his problems, Curtis had his good side. Corcoran wrote a summary at the end of the school year calling Curtis personable and honest. She said she liked him. She saw him as a basically innocent kid who couldn't always control himself. His classroom teacher, Cooper, said Curtis was more responsive and friendly to him than the average fourth grader.

Curtis did have some quirks that could get in the way of personal relationships. He sometimes did not handle racial differences well. Twice he had lunch with a third-grade girl named Jeanne Wong. He made fun of her eyes and launched into his version of Chinese. Jeanne found it funny. Later he had a substitute teacher with Asian features. Curtis made comments about the substitute's appearance and did his Chinese routine. The substitute did not find it funny. He sat Curtis down and had a discussion but did not change Curtis's mindset.

When Curtis accompanied his class on a field trip, it did not go well. He was argumentative with the other kids and began to hit one of them with his gloves. None of the other kids would be his partner. They told him to shut up and called him names. Despite it all, Curtis maintained a healthy self-image. As part of the year-end evaluations in preparation for middle school, Curtis was given a series of yes/no questions. Curtis indicated that he was smart, good looking, happy, well behaved in school, had many friends, and had nice hair. He denied that his classmates made fun of him, or that he caused trouble to his family. The evaluator commented, "It is doubtful how realistic Curtis is."

As the school year ended, Corcoran wrote down some tips for the Orono middle school that Curtis would be attending for fifth grade. Some were practical: Give him a locker with a key because numbers will likely frustrate him. Give him a closed desk to keep his things in because he is very possessive. Schedule regular times for hand washing.

Others grappled directly with the dark underside of Prader-Willi syndrome: Closely supervise him in the cafeteria because he is always hungry and has low resistance to eating any food he sees, even on the floor or in garbage cans. Be very consistent with your limits. Don't get involved in arguing with him because he will never admit to being wrong. If you need to remove him, take an arm and bend it behind him and push enough so he can feel it. Have an isolated, stimulus-free room for time-outs. Have a male available for very big tantrums.

When the school year ended, the Schumann Elementary staff exchanged good-byes with Curtis. He was a kid they were unlikely to forget. Some of them also might have said a silent prayer for the staff at the Orono middle school.

Fifteen

A Home of Their Own

If Daniel Neason had been the poster boy for PWS, and Curtis Deterling a struggling understudy, then Lisa Wett was somewhere back in the chorus. Marge and Dick kept her in special schools for the handicapped, except for a brief period in junior high when she was mainstreamed. That was a disaster, Marge later told a reporter. Lisa couldn't stop thinking about food.

Lisa's IQ tested at 69, which was conveniently just below the threshold for mental retardation. That made things easier for Marge and Dick—they were able to get the state to pay for Lisa to attend special schools. Lisa's IQ was probably higher, but Marge had a trick for making sure Lisa didn't test too high. She would bring along a bag of M&Ms when Lisa took an IQ test and tell Lisa that as soon as she was done she could have them. That got her racing through the questions "pretty darn fast," as Marge put it.

Marge called Lisa one of the "sunshine kids" because her behavior problems were less severe overall. Still, she could be a handful. She would badger Marge, "Can I have more food? Can I have this? Can I have treat?" She would sneak quietly from her bedroom at night on her tiny feet, foraging for food. One night she found a bag of cookies and brought it back to her bedroom to eat. She hid the empty bag under her pillow and went back to sleep. The family noticed it in the morning, but Lisa denied any culpability.

"No way. I did not eat those."

"But it was under your pillow!"

"Well, someone else put it there."

Finally Dick and Marge lashed a bungee cord to her bedroom door to lock her in at night.

Marge could feel herself burning out in 1979, when Lisa was fourteen. The strain was becoming too much for the family. Marge felt guilty, thinking that she wasn't giving enough either to her other kids or to Lisa. She worried especially about Andrew, her youngest. Once Marge got active with the local Minnesota Prader-Willi group that Gene founded, she discovered that others were already working on what seemed like the answer to her problems: a group home designed especially for people with PWS. Karen Virnig, another mother of a child with PWS, had taken the lead on the group home project, aided by Fausta and others. Fausta also saw that as a potential solution for Curtis, when he got older.

By fall 1980, the home—named Oakwood—was ready to open. It just needed final official approval. Oakwood would have room for fifteen people with Prader-Willi syndrome. Lisa was the youngest on the list, but Marge had no doubts about sending her there. She told a reporter, "There are people who ask how we can consider placing our daughter in a home, but they don't really understand Prader-Willi. If she knows she's going to get food and be entertained, she'll be happy. If the neighbors offered to feed her twice as much as we do, she would be on their doorstep with a suitcase."

Around this time, spring 1981, while waiting for Oakwood to open, Marge let loose in the pages of *The Gathered View*. She complained that well-meaning but clueless professionals expected people with PWS to fit into existing programs and group homes, and to work toward independence.

Marge was having none of it: "I feel their compulsions relate to their brain defect and are not controllable in the usual manner. These young people have very concrete (fixed) ideas and cannot be threatened with punishment, denials or that type of regulation because it just doesn't work. Their stubbornness and manipulative behavior is as much a part of their make-up as breathing. PW people cannot achieve independence because they cannot control their compulsive behaviors." One thing that did work, though, was being positive: "They need a very structured program. But they do respond to praise. You can get a lot of mileage out of a smile or a hug."

Finally, on September 1, 1981, Oakwood opened its doors, and Lisa moved in. She was sixteen. As Marge had predicted, Lisa was happy at Oakwood. Lisa told a reporter, "I like the activities. There are nice things. We go to movies." There was an exercise room and a rec room with a TV set, VCR, and pool table. Lisa had her own TV and VCR in her room, stuffed animals covering her bed, and her craft work on the walls. Lisa also enjoyed regular visits home, where she would play cards, visit with her nephews and nieces, take walks, and sneak the occasional candy. When she was no longer on constant guard duty, Marge found it easier to enjoy Lisa.

Marge had found her mission: to help other families find a similar solution. Her main ally was Dorothy Thompson, the director of a residential facility for the developmentally disabled in Minnesota. Dorothy had noticed that of the facility's 103 clients, the two with Prader-Willi syndrome took up 90 percent of her staff's time. Dorothy became convinced that people with PWS needed separate group homes. She became the main advisor to the mothers who were trying to get Oakwood up and running.

After Oakwood opened, Dorothy and Marge began traveling the country, meeting with local PWS chapters and helping them open group homes in their states. The number of Prader-Willi group homes slowly began to rise, as small bands of parents wrestled with logistics and red tape. By 1987 there were twenty-one Prader-Willi homes across the nation. Marge also threw herself into organizing the annual conferences and fielding phone calls, giving information and advice to parents and professionals. Under Sam and Marge's leadership, PWSA was growing nicely, reaching 1,350 members by 1984.

That year, PWSA finally managed to land the big one: Andrea Prader agreed to come to the 1984 conference, to be held in Minneapolis in June. Prader had become the director of the Kinderspital, the Zurich children's hospital where he and his colleagues had discovered Prader-Willi syndrome. He was considered one of the preeminent pediatricians in the world.

The Italians would bring their children with PWS to him as if he were the pope; the children would kneel before him while he put his hand on their heads. A junior colleague once asked him why he did it. He said, "If that's what they need, that's what I'll do!" Nor were Americans above a little Prader-worship. In 1981 Prader visited the United States, stopping in Iowa City to see Zellweger. A local parent got to meet Prader, and wrote about it for *The Gathered View*: "He is a very warm and friendly person and I only wish all of you could have had the same opportunity. We were allowed to ask questions and visit with him. It was a day to remember!"

For Prader and America, the admiration went both ways. On that same trip, Zellweger and some colleagues took Prader out to a steak house. Prader, a small man, ordered the largest steak on the menu. He dug into it, ignoring the side dishes. One of the Americans said to him: "You don't have to eat that whole thing. We just thought we'd show you what a good steak was like." Prader replied, "You don't understand. I have never eaten a steak this good or this size, and I plan to eat every bit of it. If I do nothing else, I will eat this steak."

When he arrived in Minneapolis for the PWSA conference, he visited Oakwood. The residents took him by the arm and insisted he see each of their bedrooms. It seemed to Marge that Prader was overwhelmed by the conference—the total attendance was more than four hundred—and the scope of what PWSA and the local chapters were doing.

When it came time to give his speech, Prader acknowledged a paradox: "It is impressive to see how much progress in medical knowledge and in practical management has occurred in the twenty-eight years since my colleagues Dr. Alex Labhart, Dr. Heinrich Willi, and I have given the first short description of this syndrome. On the other hand, we realize painfully how much we do not yet know and how little we can do."

He admitted his own frustration at having been unable to make further discoveries about the syndrome: "The parents expected more from me. They wanted me to explain the cause and wanted treatment, which would make these children completely normal. I always had to disappoint them."

He credited parents for teaching him about managing the syndrome: "I have frequently admired mothers who were able to manage, or to keep to certain limits, the obesity problem of their child with this syndrome, and I have learned from them, for instance, how to give food only as a reward for some physical exercise."

And, as Marge had suspected, he said he was "deeply impressed" by PWSA: "You were the first Prader-Willi syndrome association in the world, bringing together parents, doctors, other health workers and teachers. Why are you ahead of us Europeans with your association? It is one of the most admirable qualities of American people to develop very powerful private initiative; to have a strong will to help each other, not to be ashamed to have a so-called abnormal child and to go public in support of these children. It is a great experience for me to see what you are doing."

Gene and Fausta felt satisfaction and some pride after Prader spoke. The great man had blessed their brainchild. Or perhaps PWSA had blessed Prader? But Gene and Fausta couldn't enjoy the warm feelings for long. Curtis was in middle school, and he was struggling.

Sixteen

CURTIS MOVES OUT

Curtis tried to have a good attitude in middle school and do what he was supposed to do. It started well enough. He needed only two time-outs over his first three months. Fausta told the staff she was very satisfied with Curtis's progress.

The staff developed three crisp goals for Curtis:

1. Curtis will follow directions without arguing.
2. Curtis will return to tasks after time-out.
3. Curtis will be polite and considerate of peers and adults.

One year later the school reported that Curtis was following directions without arguing only 40 percent of the time, and was polite and considerate of others only 50 percent of the time. The following year the school had a more modest goal: "Curtis will follow directions without arguing 60 percent of the time." Even that goal was not met. The promising start had fizzled out.

There were days that Curtis exploded, for example, when returning to the school after participating in Special Olympics. He had been given some cookies at the event, and his management aide, Martha Brown, was holding onto them. He wanted to eat at least some of them, but Brown told him he couldn't have them until the school day was over. He told her she was wrong. She told him to go to the resource room. He lunged at her. It took three men to drag him to a time-out.

As in elementary school, the staff experimented with how much to expose Curtis to the mainstream kids. They put him in mainstream science for sixth grade, then revoked it in seventh grade. He was in mainstream art, but Brown had to handle the X-Acto knife for him.

Curtis had habits that made it hard for him to get along with his peers. An eighth-grade teacher reported: "Curtis has trouble keeping quiet at times and just letting a subject drop. He will keep talking and talking. Often the other children in the class will tell Curtis to be quiet because they are tired of hearing him talk."

Gene and Fausta met periodically with the staff. They shared a phrase they used with Curtis at home, "I can't hear you when you're shouting." Gene kept telling them: Curtis can't be pushed. Less stick, more carrot.

Midway through eighth grade, Curtis's case manager had a phone conference with Fausta to tell her things were not going well. Curtis was refusing to do assignments or take spelling tests. He had told her he was "far above the crowd" and that she was only insulting him with her demands. It was looking increasingly as if this would be the final year for Curtis in a mainstream school setting. Fausta was disappointed. She told the case manager that Curtis was so looking forward to going to the neighborhood high school.

By the end of eighth grade, it was official: Curtis would no longer remain in the Orono public school district. The school district decided he needed a more controlled environment. District 287 agreed to place him in a classroom for kids with significant cognitive and behavioral challenges, located at St. Louis Park High School. Instead of going to the Orono high school, less than two miles from his home, he would have to travel sixteen miles each way. The report from the Orono staff put the best face on it. It said Curtis would benefit from a classroom structured to his specific behavior problems. But the new classroom was even less adept at dealing with Curtis's behavioral issues than the Orono schools had been.

The power struggles escalated. By March 1987, Curtis was at an impasse with his teacher at St. Louis Park. He refused to go back to school as long as he was losing privileges. The teacher refused to restore the privileges until Curtis apologized. Curtis refused to apologize.

A compromise was worked out, and Curtis returned to school. But things were slipping out of control. Curtis was gaining weight and acting out. He was increasingly creative in his attempts to get extra food. Given the slightest opportunity, he would shoplift food. His big sister, Sara, found a heap of candy wrappers under the couch while she was vacuuming.

He got hold of Fausta's checkbook and made a surreptitious call to a local pizza parlor for six large pizzas. He made the check out for fifty dollars and in place of a signature he wrote, "For a party." He told them, "I'll leave the check on the back of the car. You don't have to bother coming to the door. Just leave the pizzas there." His plan was thwarted when someone at the pizza place got suspicious and called back, and Fausta answered the phone.

In May of that year, when he was sixteen years old, Curtis came up with a direct solution to the locks Gene and Fausta had put on the kitchen cabinets. He waited until the middle of the night, got Gene's saw, and began sawing his way into the cabinets to get at the food. Gene had had enough. He decided that they had to place Curtis in a residential facility.

The logical choice would have been Oakwood. Fausta had worked to get it opened for just this scenario. But Curtis refused to go there. Curtis knew Oakwood well, having visited with Fausta many times over the years, and he didn't think it was for him. He told the director of Oakwood, "I don't need that. I'm not like those people."

It was Dorothy Thompson who found a solution: Laura Baker Services, in Northfield, sixty miles to the south. Laura Baker served a range of clients with developmental disabilities. Dorothy told Fausta she knew some people there and that they could probably handle Curtis. Curtis's reaction was: "No, no, no, I'm not going to do that, I'm not going to go." Gene told him, "You're going to go Curtis, that's it." But Curtis remained opposed. Gene finally realized what the obstacle might be. He said, "Look, Curtis, we're going to buy you a nice big trunk so we can put all your stuff in there."

Curtis thought about that a while and he said, "Okay. Can I pick out the trunk?" From that point on Curtis was on board. Curtis moved in to Laura Baker on June 7, 1987. He was sixteen years old, five feet two inches tall, and 176 pounds. With a body mass index (BMI) of 32, he was officially obese, though not morbidly obese. For all of Gene and Fausta's efforts, Curtis was struggling.

Lots of other people were also struggling with Prader-Will syndrome. Schools didn't know what to do. Doctors didn't know what to do. Maybe it was nothing more than a ragtag group of food-obsessed, cognitively and behaviorally challenged people. Maybe there was no larger lesson to be learned, no larger pattern.

The geneticists were as frustrated as everyone else. The exciting discovery of a microdeletion on chromosome 15 had given way to confusion. As more data came in, it looked like up to 50 percent of people with PWS did not have the microdeletion. So was PWS caused by a defect on chromosome 15, or wasn't it?

Seventeen

THE GREAT GENETICS MYSTERY

Sherlock Holmes once said, "When you have eliminated the impossible, whatever remains, however improbable, must be the truth." Three theories about the relationship between chromosome 15 and Prader-Willi syndrome were investigated in the 1980s. Each was shown to be, well, not impossible, but highly unlikely. At the end of the decade, a fourth theory emerged—one so improbable that the geneticists could hardly conceive it. And that fourth theory turned out to be the truth.

The first theory was that if you diagnosed Prader-Willi syndrome carefully, making sure that all the major symptoms were present, then every person with PWS would have the chromosome 15 microdeletion. According to this theory, the supposed cases of Prader-Willi syndrome with normal-looking chromosomes were just misdiagnoses—people who did not really have PWS. Several PWS researchers subscribed to this theory. Prader also leaned this way.

But Suzanne Cassidy, a young MD with a specialty in genetics, wasn't so sure. She had become fascinated with PWS when Vic Riccardi showed up at the University of Washington in summer 1980 to talk about his lab's big discovery of a microdeletion in Prader-Willi syndrome. Cassidy connected with Vanja Holm's clinic and got a crash course in PWS. She got her first professorship at the University of Connecticut and wrote a long paper on PWS that got her recognized as an expert. She collected a group of patients with PWS whom she had carefully diagnosed herself. She worked with a laboratory-based geneticist, using the best practices to determine whether her thirteen patients had the chromosome 15 microdeletion. The result: nine had the deletion, four didn't. Theory one was out. There really were people with genuine Prader-Willi syndrome who did not have the chromosome 15 microdeletion.

The second theory was that the chromosome 15 microdeletion did not cause PWS. According to this theory, the deletion was a red herring. Hans Zellweger pushed this idea at scientific conferences and in an article in *The Gathered View*. He emphasized a small number of atypical cases that did not fit the usual patterns. But Zellweger's view did not attract many followers. It just seemed obvious to nearly everyone else that the large number of Prader-Willi cases with the deletion, and the absence of the deletion in normal humans, made it overwhelmingly likely that the deletion did cause the syndrome.

The third theory was the most attractive. It was Ledbetter's view as well as Cassidy's view that every patient with PWS had a deletion. It was just that some of the deletions were too small to be detected with current techniques. This was a reasonable extrapolation from the past, as new techniques had steadily increased the knowledge of the genetics of PWS. The only problem was, the smaller deletions weren't showing up. Ledbetter kept trying to find them, using the best techniques available. He couldn't find smaller deletions in PWS, although he did find them in another syndrome.

A younger researcher named Tim Donlon tried to find them using an even newer technique, molecular probes. Donlon was a backpacker from Oregon who had an undergraduate degree in biology and found his way, largely by accident, to a cytogenetics lab at the Oregon Health and Science University. The head of the lab was Ellen Magenis, a well-known geneticist who gave her students freedom to pursue projects that interested them. Donlon became fascinated by the new molecular probe techniques.

The probes were bits of DNA with a unique sequence that could pick out one particular spot in the human genome. You could use them to tell with great accuracy whether a particular tiny bit of DNA was present or absent from a person's chromosomes. Donlon wanted to use probes to find smaller deletions in PWS. The hard part was developing probes for the proximal 15q region—only a few advanced labs had the expertise and the equipment, which involved lasers and fluorescence.

In 1984 Donlon got his doctorate and applied for a fellowship in the lab of Samuel Latt at Harvard. Latt had the equipment Donlon needed. When Donlon proposed developing probes for Prader-Willi syndrome, Latt responded that he had also been thinking of doing that. He hired Donlon, and two years later Donlon had his probes. But when he used them on patients with PWS, he was disappointed. The probes could not detect smaller deletions.

Theory three was looking less and less likely. Even the best new techniques could not find tiny deletions in those Prader-Willi patients without the typical microdeletion. The door was open for a fourth theory, an improbable theory, to walk through.

The first clue pointing to something truly novel was reported by another young genetics researcher in 1983. Merlin Butler decided to investigate whether the deletion in Prader-Willi syndrome occurred more often on the chromosome 15 from the mother or the chromosome 15 from the father. He got a surprisingly stark result: the deletion was on the chromosome 15 from the father in all eleven Prader-Willi patients that he studied.

The significance of this clue was not appreciated at first. For generations, geneticists had been taught that it did not matter whether a gene came from the father or the mother. And that was true for the large majority of genes. But Prader-Willi syndrome was about to teach geneticists that it wasn't true for all genes.

The second clue was uncovered in Ellen Magenis's lab, with an assist from Sam Latt's lab. Latt's lab had found three patients with visible 15q deletions who did not have Prader-Willi syndrome, including one with something called Angelman syndrome. Donlon was still close to Magenis, and he told her about the patients.

Magenis jumped on the tip. She did her own digging, and found three Angelman patients with visible 15q deletions—and oddly, the deletions looked the same as the deletions in PWS. Magenis had a reputation for solid, careful work. Her paper, published in 1987, changed the landscape. The new landscape was bewildering. Angelman syndrome had little in common with Prader-Willi syndrome. The Angelman patients had little or no speech, moved with a odd jerky gait, and laughed for no apparent reason. It was sometimes called "happy puppet syndrome" because the patients were like mute, mirthful puppets jerked about by unseen strings.

Magenis speculated that even though the deletions in the two syndromes looked the same under the microscope, they would turn out to be different when examined with molecular probes. Donlon, who had left Harvard for Stanford, was eager to prove her right. He used his probes on her three Angelman patients and compared the results with six Prader-Willi patients. The probes came back with the same answer: the deletions appeared to be the same in both PWS and Angelman syndrome.

The third clue was uncovered by another prominent geneticist—a researcher named Art Beaudet, at Baylor University in Houston. In 1987 he was working on a different genetics mystery—trying to find the gene that caused cystic fibrosis, which was known to be somewhere on chromosome 7. Unlike Prader-Willi syndrome, in which a deletion on one chromosome apparently was enough to cause the syndrome, CF was a classic recessive disorder. You needed to inherit a bad gene from both parents to get the progressive, fatal disease.

Or so it was thought, until Beaudet found a fourteen-year-old girl with CF who never should have gotten sick. Her mother was a carrier, but her father was not. She should have been fine. But she had somehow ended up with two chromosome 7s from her mother and none from her father. She got two bad genes from her mother, and came down with the deadly disease. No one had ever seen this before—two of the same number chromosome from one parent and none from the other—but a few years earlier a researcher named Eric Engel had speculated that it might happen. He had come up with a name for the phenomenon. He called it "uniparental disomy"—UPD— a scientific way of saying "two chromosomes from one parent."

The fourth and final clue was buried in a few sentences of the paper that Beaudet published on his UPD patient. He and his colleagues did a literature search and discovered that UPD might cause disease by a novel mechanism that had been found in mice. Several years earlier, researchers tried to create mice that had two genetic fathers but no mother. The fertilized eggs started to develop, but then things went wrong and the embryos were defective. The reverse experiment—two genetic mothers but no father—also led to defective embryos.

These experiments suggested that a baby mouse had to get certain genes from its father and other genes from its mother. The researchers called this novel concept "imprinting." They chose this term because it looked like some genes were marked, or imprinted, according to which parent the genes came from.

It was a suggestive mix of clues, but even Beaudet and Ledbetter—who was a co-author of Beaudet's UPD paper—did not see the answer right away. It is hard to see the unexpected. The field was left open to another young researcher, one who came a long way.

Eighteen

ONE PUZZLE SOLVED

Growing up in rural Australia, Rob Nicholls and his little brother collected and bred frogs. Sometimes they would lose track of them and then find the dried-up carcasses months or years later, in hiding places around the house. Animals fascinated Nicholls. They were a welcome distraction from the great trauma of his childhood—his big sister's illness. By age ten, she was severely anorexic and spent several years in a hospital in Melbourne. Their parents' marriage dissolved and their father disappeared from their lives.

During his second year of college at the University of Melbourne, Nicholls fell in love with genetics. He liked the idea that genetics might provide answers to medical conditions like his sister's illness. While still in college, Nicholls began working in a lab, helping with bacteria research. He discovered how much he liked digging into problems no one knew the answer to. He also found that lab work was a series of steps, like cooking. You just had to roll up your sleeves and get to it, like when he was a kid and had to cook when his mother worked late.

After finishing college in 1981, Nicholls wanted to work at one of the top labs for human genetics, which meant going to Great Britain or the United States. He was accepted at Oxford but still had to find funding. He applied for a Rhodes scholarship, but he was rejected and came out of the interview feeling that the upper-class Australians who interviewed him found him uncouth. His mother vowed to work two jobs to support him, but in the end she didn't need to—he got a different scholarship.

After earning a graduate degree from Oxford, Nicholls wanted to be at a lab doing cutting-edge work in the genetics of mental retardation, which meant going to the United States. Sam Latt accepted him at his lab at Harvard. Nicholls arrived in Cambridge planning to study the genetics of fragile X syndrome, the most common form of inherited mental impairment, but that didn't work out. Latt had another idea: Nicholls could continue the work that Tim Donlon had begun, using probes to investigate Prader-Willi syndrome. Nicholls had never heard of PWS, but he immediately found it intriguing. It was in some sense the reverse of his sister's problem—she ate too little, they ate too much.

Nicholls set to work learning how to use the probes. After presenting some preliminary work at a genetics meeting, Nicholls was approached by Merlin Butler, who had a number of Prader-Willi patients with no visible deletion. He wondered if Nicholls would like to use these patients to try to find smaller deletions with his probes. Nicholls accepted the offer. But like Donlon before him, Nicholls wasn't able to find any smaller deletions.

Now Nicholls was presented with another puzzle. A young cytogeneticist named Joan Knoll joined Latt's lab, on a mission to figure out why there seemed to be the same deletions in PWS and Angelman. Nicholls was given the job of tutoring her in how to use the probes.

Nicholls and Knoll got the same result Donlon had: both Prader-Willi and Angelman patients had deletions that appeared to be identical. Then they discovered something new and very intriguing: unlike Prader-Willi syndrome, where the deletions were always on the chromosome 15 from the father, in all four of their Angelman patients the deletions were on the chromosome 15 from the mother.

This was the critical fifth clue. The puzzle pieces slid into place in the mind of Rob Nicholls, and he had the answer to the great mystery of Prader-Willi genetics. Imprinting was the key. There were one or more genes you had to get from your father; if you didn't, you got Prader-Willi syndrome. There were also one or more genes you had to get from your mother; if you didn't, you got Angelman syndrome. All of these genes happened to be in the same region of chromosome 15, proximal 15q. If that region was deleted on your father's chromosome 15, you got PWS. If it was deleted on your mother's chromosome 15, you got Angelman.

And in the same flash, he knew why there were Prader-Willi (and presumably Angelman) patients who had no deletions. UPD was the key. If both your chromosome 15s were from your mother, you would not have certain necessary genes from your father and you would get PWS. If both your chromosome 15s were from your father, you would not have certain necessary genes from your mother and you would get Angelman syndrome. It was a beautiful explanation. Thanks to the new concepts of imprinting and UPD, all the mysteries of Prader-Willi and Angelman genetics that were baffling scientists fell away. It was so elegant, it almost had to be true.

But Nicholls and Knoll needed more evidence to convince other scientists to accept the radical new explanation. Skeptics would point out that better techniques might show that the deletions in Prader-Willi and Angelman were actually different. When Knoll and Nicholls first published, they were cautious. They wrote that their findings "suggested" that imprinting was involved, but that more work was needed. Nicholls knew what the key piece of evidence would be: he needed to show that patients with PWS who did not have a deletion had maternal UPD 15—that is, both their chromosome 15s were from their mother. Alternatively, he could have shown that Angelman patients who did not have a deletion had paternal UPD 15, but such patients were scarcer, and he already had a ready supply of Prader-Willi patients with no visible deletion, thanks to Merlin Butler.

Once Nicholls had his mental breakthrough, it seemed so obvious, and he worried that someone else would beat him to the proof. Then Sam Latt died suddenly at forty-nine years of age. Howard Hughes Medical Institute, the foundation that had been funding Latt's lab, agreed to keep the money flowing for twelve more months. After that, Nicholls would be on his own.

He was racing to prove his great theory before anyone else and before the money ran out, but the probes weren't cooperating. Nicholls was having trouble proving the parental origin of the chromosomes. Then serendipity came in the form of excessive voltage. Nicholls had set up an overnight experiment, running electricity through a gel to separate out DNA segments from one of the patients with PWS. The next morning he came back and found the gel steaming and partially melted. Somehow the voltage had been set to 150 volts—more than three times what he had meant to use. Perhaps he had forgotten to turn down the voltage the night before. Perhaps, thought Nicholls, someone had tried to sabotage his experiment.

The normal response would have been to toss out the gel and start over. But Nicholls remembered times at Oxford when a gel that was accidentally dropped on the floor and broke into pieces still yielded results. So he decided to go ahead and process his pitiful, partially collapsed gel. Other people in the lab found this funny.

The extra voltage had created a separation between two bands of DNA. That was the missing piece of evidence he was looking for, to prove that the patient with PWS had two chromosome 15s from his mother and none from his father. "Bang, there was the absolute proof," Nicholls said later.

Nicholls published his work in the November 16, 1989 issue of *Nature*, with Knoll and Butler as co-authors. They had documented a brand new disease mechanism in humans. And they had shown the world the answer to the mystery of Prader-Willi genetics. When Ledbetter and Beaudet heard about Nicholls's breakthrough, they were "kicking themselves in the butt," as Ledbetter later put it, for not having thought of it themselves. Looking back, all the clues they needed were in their own paper on the cystic fibrosis patient with UPD.

Other geneticists had a less conflicted reaction. John Opitz, who as founder of the *American Journal of Medical Genetics* had published many articles on the mysteries of PWS, said he was "surprised and delighted." He called the sequence of discoveries "one of the most gratifying in modern human genetics." Andrea Prader was pleased, too. In 1991 the seventy-one-year-old Prader said, "I am happy to be alive to witness the increasing interest in this syndrome among pediatricians and geneticists, and to see how it has become important as one of the first examples in man of the new genetic mechanisms of UPD and imprinting."

Prader's syndrome was all grown up. Now it had a clear cause: a lack of genetic material in a specific region of chromosome 15. No one could doubt anymore whether it was a real syndrome. No one could say anymore that it was all the parents' fault. The real beneficiaries were not the small number of families like the Deterlings who had been lucky enough to have their children diagnosed as babies. The real beneficiaries—once Nicholls and others came up with a laboratory test—were all the families to come. Now a simple blood draw could diagnose the syndrome in an infant. Now so many more families could know, so much earlier, what they were dealing with.

The discovery was a milestone in Rob Nicholls's life, as well. Now he had no trouble finding a job. The frog-collecting boy from rural Australia became an assistant professor at the University of Florida in Gainesville.

But despite the genetics breakthrough, practical treatments for PWS were still scarce. Knowing that people with PWS were missing one or more genes perhaps made their caregivers more sympathetic to them, but it did not provide any insight into how to manage them. Parents, teachers, group home workers—they were all trying to figure it out as they went along.

Part III

A Kind of Maturity

Ninteen

When Curtis moved into Laura Baker at age sixteen, Gene felt relief. He planned a celebratory trip to Alaska for himself and Fausta, but she did not feel like celebrating. She thought, "My own kid and I'm sending him away." Curtis had never really been apart from her. She figured she could call him every day, but the staff at Laura Baker told them no phone calls or visits for the first two weeks. This made Fausta feel even worse, like she had abandoned Curtis. Gene reassured her, "He needs to get accustomed to it." At least they could write him a letter. Fausta wrote how much they loved him, and Gene wrote how proud they were of him.

Laura Baker had been founded back in 1897. It had more than seventy live-in clients, ranging from mildly handicapped to severely developmentally disabled. Prader-Willi syndrome was relatively new to them—Curtis was one of the first. Many of the older residents lived in isolation from their families; their parents had been advised to put them in a facility and forget about them. This was not Curtis's fate. Once those initial two weeks were up, Gene and Fausta visited him often, taking him on outings and home for weekends. Still, at the outset Curtis was not thrilled with his new living situation. At a meeting to assess his first thirty days, he was argumentative and emotional, disagreeing often with his parents and the Laura Baker staff. He was still on the heavy side, at 175 pounds.

After five months at Laura Baker, he had lost 30 pounds, simply because food was better controlled in this new environment. He was taking regular showers, whereas at first, according to a November 1987 report, "it was a daily struggle to get him near water." "He is generally in a calm and contented emotional state," the report continued. "He can communicate very well and is at ease conversing with strangers as well as peers, staff and family." He did become physically aggressive at times, usually when the staff were trying to set a limit that Curtis thought unreasonable, but at a rate of just one incident a month.

Bruce Jensen, a behavioral analyst at Laura Baker who often worked with Curtis, took a liking to him. Jensen had had a difficult time in his teen years, losing both his parents by the summer after high school. After earning a college degree in music education, he gave up his plans to become a teacher, afraid he would be bad at discipline. He joined the Army instead and played the French horn in an Army band in Germany. He didn't know what to do after that. He went to stay with his sister in Northfield, and met her friend, Deana Antley, who worked at Laura Baker. Deana told him, "You ought to give this a shot."

At Laura Baker, Jensen found his place. He loved the job. And he particularly liked the clients with PWS. Jensen thought they had an effervescence—they would just sparkle when you knew them well. The degree to which they could enjoy a moment was exceptional. He enjoyed Curtis's boisterous, infectious laugh, and his sense of the absurd. Anything a ten-year-old would find funny, Curtis would find hilarious. Deana Antley also enjoyed Curtis. He would visit her in her office several times a week, with a big smile on his face and a "Hey, how are you?" He would chat about what he was up to and ask Antley about her kids, her grandkids, her dog, her Dodge van.

When his first autumn at Laura Baker came around, Curtis started attending the special education program at the local high school, Northfield High. His new management aide, Ann Strawn, was fond of "Curt," as she called him. She described him as "reasonably cooperative" with a "generally optimistic, extroverted personality." His initial defensive reaction to teasing from peers was giving way to tolerance. By the second semester, he was enjoying talking about cars and engines with the other boys during breaks between classes. And he was thinking ahead. Strawn wrote, "He has decided to become a pediatrician and would like to arrange a work experience in that field!"

Sometimes Prader-Willi issues would intrude. Curtis always fell asleep when stories were read in English class. He learned some simple computer programming—using a language called Logo to make images—but he got frustrated and angry when he couldn't make the images as good as his imagination. He dropped the class. He was not keeping up academically in English or math.

There were problems at Laura Baker, too. One day in October during his second year there, a staff member told Curtis to change the sheets on his bed. Curtis said he didn't need to. The staff member insisted, calling the bedding a health hazard. He gave Curtis three warnings, but Curtis still refused to do it. The staff member went into Curtis's room and began changing the sheets. Curtis, outraged, grabbed the sheets from him. The staff member dropped him to the floor and restrained him while two other staff members made the bed. Then they marched Curtis to the director's office for a time-out. On the way there Curtis struck out five times, bending his glasses in the process. Curtis told the lead staff member he was not only going to kill him, but fire him, too.

Curtis spent two more years at Northfield High. Ann Strawn was no longer his management aide. His behaviors deteriorated. A report at the end of his second year stated: "He makes noises and laughs inappropriately. He has become more insistent in stating his opinions and is more aggressive towards students and staff, both verbally and physically. The aggressive and noncompliant behavior continue for longer periods of time and appear to give Curtis satisfaction."

Still, Curtis attended Northfield High's graduation ceremony and received a certificate. Then, ready or not, it was time for him to enter the world of work. But how? Would Curtis work at a sheltered workshop for the developmentally disabled, doing simple tasks? Or would he, with assistance, work in the community?

Curtis's team decided to pursue both options. Curtis initially spent most of his time at a sheltered workshop affiliated with Laura Baker. He also got a job in the community, doing maintenance work at Northfield schools—picking up trash and pulling weeds. Then he got a more exciting job: working at the Ice Arena, where he swept the bleachers and floors, cleaned glass, and cleaned bathrooms.

Going to real work sites meant having to follow real-world rules. These were spelled out in a written contract designed especially for Curtis.

He was expected to:

Dress appropriately.
Be on time.
Follow directions without discussion.
Stop being inappropriate when told to.
Not constantly talk with his job coach.
Leave the work site immediately if asked to because of inappropriate behavior.

There were consequences for noncompliance—a series of warnings, which, if ignored, would lead to losing a half hour of pay. If that didn't get Curtis under control, he would be returned to Laura Baker. If he were returned three times, he would lose the job.

The clear expectations helped. Before the written contract was developed, Curtis was in danger of being booted from the Ice Arena after working there only a few weeks. After the written contract was put in place, he managed to keep working there from November all the way through the following June.

Curtis had shown that he could handle maintenance jobs, with a lot of support. Now his team had a more ambitious goal: to prepare Curtis for jobs in the community where he would be interacting with the public. To get him ready, they enrolled him at Dakota County Technical Center, where he took classes on job-related skills.

They tried Curtis in the office of a veterinarian, Dr. Garley. Curtis loved animals, so it seemed like the ideal worksite. Curtis's responsibilities included cleaning, doing laundry, sterilizing instruments, sterilizing and lining animal cages, and walking animals.

The first problem was his wandering fingers. The job coach caught Curtis stealing candy from the secretary's desk and made Curtis apologize to her. Another time, the job coach caught him with an animal bone treat in his pocket.

The second problem was his overactive mouth. He would bombard customers with questions about their animals and why they had brought them in. He argued with the secretary and with Garley. Once when Garley was putting a cat to sleep, Curtis told him it was a mistake and said, "No wonder why people say he's a bad doctor." The job coach made him apologize.

The evaluator concluded that Curtis "certainly has the ability to complete a number of entry level tasks. At times, he can work very appropriately within community based settings. . . . On other occasions, Curtis requires constant behavioral intervention due to behaviors such as arguing, crying and theft." Her conclusion: "Until behavior is more stabilized, I feel a sheltered workshop would be the most appropriate placement for Curtis."

Despite his difficulties with work and his behavioral problems, Curtis was getting a lot of enjoyment out of his life. He loved to read, work on jigsaw puzzles, play computer games, and play word-find games. He enjoyed Scrabble. He liked to watch TV, especially *The Simpsons*, wildlife shows, professional wrestling, and police action shows. He especially liked being outdoors: walking, swimming, cross-country skiing, fishing, and boating.

At Laura Baker there were special events, including a family fun day in August, a fall dance, and a big Halloween party. In Northfield, there were the Defeat of Jesse James Days every September and summer concerts on Bridge Square, as well as the community swimming pool, the local movie theater, and the library. Curtis had a buddy from a local college who would visit him. Another college group came and did a multiweek workshop on how to be a clown.

Curtis also enjoyed being helpful around his parents' house. He would mow the lawn, weed, shovel snow, vacuum, and set the table. And he especially enjoyed collecting. He collected books, magazines, puzzles, games, wildlife cards, miniature cars and trucks, computer games, and stuffed animals. His room overflowed with his collections.

Despite the bumps, it was a promising start for Curtis, living away from his family for the first time. Still, Gene and Fausta wanted more. They wished Curtis could be better behaved overall, so he could do more challenging and satisfying work and get more out of his leisure time. They wondered if perhaps some medication could help.

Twenty

A Drug For PWS Behaviors?

Just as the Deterlings were searching for something to improve Curtis's behavior, a new drug came along: Prozac. It was touted in a short article in the March 1991 issue of *The Gathered View*. The article said that unlike earlier behavior medications, Prozac was non-sedating and did not promote weight gain. It was an antidepressant, but the article said it could also help with obsessive-compulsive behavior, kleptomania, and obesity, and that "it has been successfully used for some of our children." The next issue had more exciting news about Prozac: it had helped a person with Prader-Willi syndrome lose 22 pounds over six months, and had decreased her compulsion to pull out and eat her hair.

The Deterlings convinced Curtis's regular doctor to try him on Prozac. Curtis began taking the lowest dose, 20 mg a day, on February 21, 1991. The article in the newsletter said it would take two to four weeks to see any results, but in Curtis the effect was instantaneous. He was calmer, happier, laughing more. In a year-end summary, Bruce Jensen noted that before starting on Prozac, Curtis was verbally aggressive during 22 percent of the time periods charted, whereas after starting the drug, that figure dropped to 10 percent. There was a similar decrease in disruptive behavior, minutes in time-out, and the need for manual restraint. Finally, there was a medicine that helped with the most difficult parts of Prader-Willi syndrome.

But it didn't last. By fall 1991 Curtis had returned to his baseline level of misbehavior. His doctor doubled the dose to 40 mg per day. The increase had no effect. Now Gene and Fausta had a dilemma. Should they go back to 20 mg, or increase the dose again? As they were mulling it over, Curtis started having more explosive outbursts. They decided to up the dose to 60 mg per day.

The higher dose backfired. Curtis became more agitated. To Fausta, it seemed he was having tantrums over everything, like a little child, and being verbally aggressive. He would tell her, "I'll do what I want. You can't stop me." The doctor dropped the Prozac back to 20 mg and started Curtis on an anti-anxiety drug called Buspar. This combination seemed to work pretty well, but after riding the drug roller coaster with Curtis, his parents were feeling nauseous. They decided that a psychiatrist should oversee Curtis's behavior medications.

On January 20, 1993 Curtis had his first appointment at the Southern Cities Community Health Clinic in Faribault. He began regular visits with a psychiatrist, Frederick Ferron, and a pharmacist, Cynthia Kern. Over the next year and a half Ferron and Kern tinkered with his medications.

When Curtis seemed to be doing worse, they substituted Zoloft for Prozac (Zoloft is another so-called SSRI drug, in the same family as Prozac). Then they went on the same roller coaster ride that Curtis had been on with Prozac. They started at 25 mg of Zoloft and soon increased it to 50 mg. Curtis was happier and had fewer outbursts. When Curtis started having more verbal outbursts, they increased the Zoloft to 100 mg. Curtis's behaviors deteriorated, and he began picking at his scalp with greater intensity.

Kern noted, "Zoloft has not seemed to be consistently useful, from doses of 25 to 100 mg." They decreased the dose and then dropped it completely. She and Ferron considered other meds: Depakote? Fenfluramine? Propranolol? Then they threw up their hands and went back to Zoloft. They were swayed by Curtis's opinion: he thought Zoloft had been useful. The Laura Baker staff were not so sure.

At the next clinic visit, in July 1994, everything seemed good. Curtis had had no physical aggression and only one verbal outburst since restarting Zoloft. He talked excitedly about the upcoming PWSA conference in Atlanta, which he was going to attend with his parents. Curtis loved going to PWSA conferences. There was a young adult program with activities, arts and crafts, and outings. There was the Saturday night banquet with the big dance at the end. And there was his girlfriend, Page, whose mother, Marilyn, had attended the very first PWSA conference.

Page Bintz was born in 1971, like Curtis. She was diagnosed with PWS when she was six years old and already weighed 75 pounds. After the diagnosis Marilyn began working with the Prader-Willi nutritionist in Sacramento, California, near their home in Davis. Soon she got Page down to an age-appropriate 43 pounds. For a while Page's weight was well managed. She and Curtis had met at an earlier conference, and had decided they were boyfriend and girlfriend. This mostly meant they would dance together at the conference banquet. They saw each other only once a year, but they both looked forward to it.

Things had not gone well for Page since the last conference. She had always had a compulsion to take things that weren't hers, but after she turned eighteen she became more brazen. She was twice caught breaking into other people's houses and was sent to the Stockton Development Center, a psychiatric facility. No special allowances were made for her oversized appetite, and Page took full advantage. Eventually she had around 250 pounds packed onto her four-foot-eight-inch frame.

When Curtis saw her at the conference, he didn't recognize her. She had gained about 100 pounds since the last conference. He could not believe this was his Page. Adding to his shock, he had learned the day before that another friend of his with PWS had died. Curtis became withdrawn and lethargic, and he had difficulty sleeping. He refused to attend the banquet and the dance. Gene blamed Curtis's behavior medications. He stopped giving him Zoloft and Buspar, and instead he shared some of his Halcion prescription with Curtis, to help him sleep.

Gene and Fausta decided to continue with their plan to spend a week on Cape Cod after the conference. They had gone there before and Curtis had loved it. But on the Cape, Curtis got worse. He could not remember anything about the conference he had just attended. He asked repetitive questions, was fearful and guilty, and apologized incessantly. He continued to have trouble sleeping and got increasingly agitated. He said to Fausta, "I want to bite you." He kept coming toward her. He looked serious about it.

Gene had had enough of Curtis's "silly talk," as he called it. He and Fausta took Curtis to the emergency room at the hospital in Hyannis. The emergency room doctor prescribed a cocktail of three drugs for Curtis: Haldol, an antipsychotic; Ativan, for anxiety; and Benadryl, as a sedative and to counteract possible side effects from the Haldol. The doctor also prescribed a second antipsychotic, Mellaril. The medications had a powerful effect on Curtis. He became catatonic—drooling, staring, and not responding, like a zombie. They had to put him in a wheelchair to get him through the airport and back home.

Once home they took him straight to the hospital. The doctor told them, "He's overmedicated. There's nothing else you can do. Just take him back home." The next day Curtis was at least coherent, but still in bad shape. Gene and Fausta took him to his regular psychiatric clinic. The psychiatrist noted that Curtis was drooling and disoriented, had poor eye contact, and kept saying he felt guilty for killing his dog and hurting his parents (neither of which was true). He also was

clinging to Fausta. The psychiatrist recommended hospital-
izing Curtis to rule out an organic cause for what she called
his "acute confusional state."

Curtis spent a week at the psychiatric unit at Fairview
Riverside Hospital. The doctors couldn't find any organic
cause for his delirium. They put him back on Zoloft, Buspar,
and Ativan. He did at least sleep through his last two nights in
the hospital, but overall his hospitalization was a very negative
experience. He was put in an isolation room for acting out. His
brother, Evan, came to visit him and was outraged to see Curtis
locked up. He insisted that Curtis be discharged, and Gene and
Fausta agreed.

Curtis spent four days at home and then returned to Laura
Baker. He was not well. He paced during the day and slept very
poorly at night. He clung to the staff, wanting to hug and kiss
them as much as eighty times in one hour. He skipped meals
and was incontinent. He kept saying things like, "What did I
do wrong?" and "How did I frighten you?"

What most saddened Bruce Jensen was the loss of bowel
control. One time he found Curtis covered in his own feces and
completely unresponsive. The Curtis he'd known—the socia-
bility, the sense of pride—seemed to be gone.

Jensen searched for a place that could help. He finally
found one about an hour's drive from Laura Baker: Mount
Olivet Rolling Acres, which served people with developmental disabilities. It offered something called the Special
Services Program, a forty-five-day residential program for
people in crisis—people who needed a calm environment and

focused attention from nurses, counselors, psychologists, and psychiatrists.

Curtis was admitted to Mount Olivet on August 17, 1994, and stayed there for the next seven weeks. In his first week he had many instances of insecurity, disorientation, and perseverative speech (repeatedly saying things like "What did I do wrong?" "Can I talk to my mother now?" or "How did I frighten you?"). By the fourth week he had far less of each. He was able to enjoy some of the activities, like shooting baskets in the gymnasium. Fausta thought it was a great place for Curtis.

In part, his progress was due to better psychiatric care. The psychiatrist at Mount Olivet continued Curtis on Risperdal, an antipsychotic, which Curtis had started taking a few days before his admission. But he also added drugs to counteract the side effects of the antipsychotic medications, which included incontinence, drooling, loss of eye contact, and lethargy.

The Mount Olivet staff concluded that Curtis had experienced a psychotic episode brought on by the stress of his girlfriend's massive weight gain and his friend's death, combined perhaps with a mood disorder, and made worse by all the side effects of the Haldol and Mellaril given to him in the emergency room at the Cape Cod hospital.

Curtis returned to Laura Baker and continued to heal. Bruce Jensen was glad to have Curtis back but was disturbed by what had been lost. Curtis didn't have the same belly laugh anymore. He was functional, but flatter. Jensen blamed the antipsychotic medications.

Gene and Fausta were eager to get Curtis off Risperdal. They thought it sedated him. By early January 1995 they had convinced Kern and Ferron to discontinue it. Off antipsychotic medications for the first time in four months, Curtis had a hard time functioning—he was obsessive and very ritualistic, had difficulty completing tasks, and got upset easily. At the next visit Kern recommended restarting Risperdal, but Curtis was opposed. As an alternative, Kern suggested trying a newer SSRI, Luvox, to replace the Zoloft.

On Luvox, Curtis's functioning improved somewhat, but there were a lot of ups and downs. Ferron and Kern tinkered with the dosage of Luvox, but there did not seem to be a clear relationship between Curtis's functioning and his medications. In May 1995 Ferron wrote in his notes, "This is obviously a complicated case."

Gene concluded that for Curtis, less was better than more. The right medications, in the right dosages, might help, but they were certainly not a cure-all. The stresses of life—some unavoidable, some due to a poorly structured living environment—were the most important factor. The Deterlings were not the only ones learning these lessons. PWSA was also increasingly focused on the nitty-gritty of coping with the difficult behaviors of the Prader-Willi population.

Twenty-One

A New Frankness

In 1980 Janalee Tomaseski was a single mother raising three children. She had a master's degree in social work from Washington University in St. Louis, and had worked with child abuse victims and in hospices. Then she met a single father, Al Heinemann, who was raising a six-year-old daughter, Sarah, and a seven-year-old son with Prader-Willi syndrome, Matt. Janalee and Al fell in love and married. In 1981 they attended their first PWSA conference, in Boca Raton, and met a number of adolescents with PWS. That night Al cried in Janalee's arms. Until then he had clung to the hope that Matt would outgrow his condition.

When they got back from the conference, the first thing they did was lock up the food. To their surprise, Matt seemed relieved. The next thing they did was get active. Together they started the first Missouri chapter of PWSA in 1982. Janalee also began writing. Her first project was a children's book she wrote with Sarah about having a sibling with PWS, called *Sometimes I'm Mad, Sometimes I'm Glad.*

Her first major piece—about the chronic grief of having a mentally disabled child—was published in the July 1984 issue of *The Gathered View.* In 1988, PWSA published its most ambitious book yet: *Management of Prader-Willi Syndrome.* The editors asked Janalee to write a chapter from a parent's perspective. The result was the most realistic picture yet of what it took to deal with the syndrome. Janalee shared food tricks, which included spreading Matt's food out to look bigger on the plate and bulking up with low-calorie garnishes. She admitted that they let Matt and Sarah eat in front of the TV, to distract Matt and give her and Al a little break. They hid food in their bedroom so they wouldn't have to eat in front of Matt. Janalee wrote, "We lock ourselves in the bedroom—for more than sex."

Janalee wrote that parents dealing with PWS have kept secret "the true tragedy of PWS, the serious behavior problems," perhaps out of shame, perhaps out of fear that their child's misbehavior reflected an inability to parent. She shared tricks that worked with Matt. Setting rules ahead of time and being consistent. Giving him a small piece of candy at bedtime if he had been good all day. Giving him a small toy if he managed five days in a row without crying at school.

When Matt started to lose it, Janalee and Al had to learn that talking it out did not work. Instead they sent him to his room until he could discuss things calmly. At first Matt would kick, scream, and tear his room apart. Anything he wrecked was later removed and not replaced. If the situation got too intense, one of them would tell Matt that if he could not settle down within five minutes, he would get only a small sandwich for dinner. As his room got barer, Matt got better, and lost a few pounds, too.

Fortunately, there was more to it than managing tantrums. Matt thrived on compliments. Janalee and Al retrained themselves to make as many positive comments as possible to Matt and to keep quiet if they couldn't say anything good.

Janalee became a PWSA board member in 1986. She and Al volunteered to lead the PWSA committee on camping and retreat facilities. As Janalee's presence on the board grew, people—including Gene and Fausta—realized that she was more than just a good writer; she was a leader.

As the 1980s drew to a close, the decade-long era of Sam and Marge was ending. The first to go was Sam. Some on the board had tired of his talkative leadership style. Starting with the July 1989 newsletter, Sam's "President's Message" was no longer on the front page. In the January 1990 issue the board announced a new rule: presidents would serve for only three years, with the possibility of one additional three-year term on a two-thirds vote.

And then the inevitable: the September 1990 newsletter announced that Sam would be resigning at the end of the year. Sam stormed out of the board meeting when he realized what was going on. But he reconciled himself to his fate, writing in the newsletter that a new president was needed to bring the organization to a higher level. He concluded, "I was once told that the most important responsibility of an executive is to identify the incompetent and fire them. Therefore, having tendered my resignation to the Board, I fire me! Remember—blame Sam. Then go do it right."

Sam's final sentence to the members was as wordy and heartfelt as Sam himself: "Only through knowledgeable parents and not uncommonly private evaluations will our Prader-Willi language and learning-disabled children receive the education and social integration they need to survive and reduce behavior problems that block their progress through a world they seldom understand and that certainly doesn't understand them."

To no one's surprise, the board chose Janalee as the new president. Also to no one's surprise, Marge and Janalee did not co-exist for long. Three months after Janalee was named the new president, Marge announced her resignation. As with Sam, Marge's personality quirks had rubbed some board members the wrong way over her long tenure. She could be undiplomatic. She had resisted the board's attempt to push the organization in a more professional direction. Marge wanted to keep doing things the old, cheap way, using black-and-white handouts instead of color brochures, to keep the informational material as affordable as possible.

Sam and Marge had shepherded the organization through tremendous growth. The membership grew from around three hundred in 1980 to some sixteen hundred in 1990, as the annual budget grew from $12,700 to $105,000 and the number of Prader-Willi group homes across the United States increased from one to twenty-six. And that was not all Sam had done. Although others would lead PWSA from here, everyone would benefit from something Sam had done, back at the start of his presidency.

Twenty-Two

A Medicine For PWS

Sam Beltran was not a man to complain, although life gave him ample opportunities. He had a quick grin and an easy manner. He would talk your ear off, then pick it up from the floor and keep talking to it.

He was born in Wisconsin to a Filipino immigrant and a mother of German descent. He had a thing for fair-skinned girls. His first love was Janet, of Norwegian ancestry. They dated all through college, as he completed his pre-med courses and was admitted to medical school. The night before graduation Janet broke up with him, saying she didn't want to marry a doctor. Four days after that he went on a blind date and met Elizabeth, another Scandinavian. Two years later, in 1952, they married and had three children over the next five years. Sam became an anesthesiologist, with a specialty in cardiac surgery.

In 1968 he drove the whole family from Wauwatosa to Palo Alto, joining the great migration to California. Stanford hired him to be the first head of its Cardiovascular Anesthesia Service.

But Elizabeth was struggling. She began drinking heavily, and Sam didn't know how to help her. Two years after the move to California, Elizabeth caught a vicious case of Asian flu. Sam rushed her to the hospital. He thought he had had the same flu the prior week, so he convinced a doctor to drain two pints of his blood, concentrate the cells, and transfuse the blood into Elizabeth, hoping it would contain antibodies to the flu. But she died, leaving Sam with their three teenage children.

Sam buried his Lizzie in April, and married his head nurse, Linda, in August. Sam and Linda's first child, Sarah, was born a year and a half later. Sarah was tiny and hardly moved. She was diagnosed with Prader-Willi syndrome when she was three years old. None of this slowed Sam down. He kept forging ahead, assisting with surgeries and trying to care for his family, which grew to include a second daughter with Linda.

In 1981, when Sam was just beginning his long term as president of PWSA, nine-year-old Sarah, already very short, stopped growing. Sam figured Sarah could benefit from growth hormone (GH). He went to the chief of pediatrics at Stanford and said he wanted to put Sarah on GH. The chief tried to dissuade him. He told Sam that he had studied GH, and he knew it had nothing to do with the short stature of people with Prader-Willi syndrome.

Sam didn't care about the medical literature or the views of chiefs of pediatrics. He figured GH might help Sarah grow, and he wanted to try it. Period. The chief told Sam, "If you're really interested in GH, go talk to Ron Rosenfeld." Rosenfeld was a more open-minded young endocrinologist. He agreed to try Sarah on GH for one year.

Sarah started the shots in mid-1982, when she was ten years old. Over the next year, she grew four inches. She was happy about that, and proud of what she was doing. Sam and Linda were proud of her, too. It was not an easy thing, as the protocol at the time required a decent-sized needle to be jabbed right into the muscle.

Around this time, Phillip Lee, a new endocrinology fellow, joined the group at Stanford and was assigned Sarah Beltran as one of his patients. Lee continued to give GH to Sarah, and got three other kids with PWS on GH. He noticed something else: not only was the GH giving a nice boost to their height, but it seemed to be giving them more energy.

Gene and Fausta heard from Sam about Sarah's success with GH, and they were eager to try it with Curtis. The problem was that Curtis hated shots. Fausta thought it was because of all the times he'd been stuck with needles when he was a baby, back when the doctors were trying to figure out what was wrong with him. Curtis put up with the GH shots for a while, but increasingly resisted them. After a few months, Fausta and Gene gave up. Curtis did, however, gain about three inches during the short time he was treated with GH.

Phillip Lee first presented on growth hormone at the 1987 PWSA conference in Houston. No one seemed too impressed. He felt isolated at that conference, a lone endocrinologist surrounded by geneticists. He witnessed a loud discussion between Zellweger and other geneticists—this was before Nicholls's breakthrough—about which patients really had PWS. Wow, Lee thought, even they don't know what the syndrome is.

His next presentation at a PWSA conference went better. In 1991, in Lincolnwood, Illinois, he had an additional study to present, showing that GH not only gave people with PWS more height, but it also gave them more muscle and denser bones. After his presentation, Lee was taking a bus back to his hotel when two mothers recognized him. "Oh yeah," they told him, "we want our kids on GH."

Lee no longer felt so isolated, as other endocrinologists began treating their Prader-Willi patients with GH. Moris Angulo, a geneticist and endocrinologist from New York, had been treating Prader-Willi patients with GH since the mid-1980s. Growing up in El Salvador, Angulo was the fattest kid in his small town. He could relate to his short, obese PWS patients. And he found them very friendly. By 1989 he had collected data comparing the natural GH secretion of patients with and without PWS, showing that the ones with PWS didn't have the usual periodic spurts of GH release. But when he presented his data at a conference, the other endocrinologists were skeptical.

There was one doctor—whose arms were folded, blocking his name tag—who encouraged Angulo, saying the results were fascinating and he should continue his work. When the man unfolded his arms, Angulo could read the name on his tag:

Andrea Prader. Angulo "went crazy," he said later. He hugged Prader, saying, "Thank you, thank you, thank you."

Angulo published those results in 1991, and in 1996 he published another paper on the beneficial effects of long-term use of GH. Angulo was not the only young endocrinologist influenced by Prader. Urs Eiholzer, a junior colleague of Prader's from Zurich, published in 1998 on the benefits of GH in young children with PWS.

Not all the GH pioneers were endocrinologists. There was also Barbara Whitman, who had a PhD in social work and degrees or certifications in medical technology, psychiatry, epidemiology, and developmental disabilities. In 1981 she helped open a developmental clinic at Cardinal Glennon Children's Medical Center in St. Louis. In walked Janalee Heinemann, saying she wanted to start a local support group for something called Prader-Willi syndrome. Whitman said, "Sure, why not." She became fascinated with PWS, and friends with Janalee and Al. She helped them with a summer camp for PWS children; she'd bring her guitar, and Janalee and Al would bring the food. After the kids went to bed, she would hit Janalee and Al's tent for beer and cheese.

After hearing Lee talk about GH at the 1991 PWSA conference, Whitman was intrigued. She played a major role in organizing larger scale controlled studies on GH in patients with PWS. She was particularly concerned about whether GH would have behavioral effects. The one effect she did notice, anecdotally, was that the patients, especially the older ones, would get a surge of energy once they started on GH. This energy was not always well directed. One woman ran off and got married. More often, they would become cleverer about getting more food. But these were not reasons to avoid GH; it just meant parents and caregivers had to make sure they had appropriate controls in place.

Under Janalee, PWSA embraced GH. Lee was invited to join PWSA's scientific advisory board, and in 1996 he wrote PWSA's policy statement on GH treatment. Between 1997 and 1999 other endocrinologists, in Europe and the United States, published controlled studies that randomly separated kids with PWS into a treatment group and a control group. All found that the group treated with GH did much better than the untreated control group.

Then a new resistance emerged from within the Prader-Willi community. A group of professionals with a long involvement in PWS pushed back against the use of GH. They were, for the most part, behaviorists, who worked directly with the most challenging aspect of the syndrome. The struggle came to a head at the 1999 PWSA conference in San Diego.

During one discussion following a presentation on the benefits of GH, a woman in the back of the room raised her hand and said, "I don't think this is right. If you change them so they don't look like Prader-Willis, people are going to start thinking they are normal. They are not normal." Phillip Lee was moderating the discussion. As he thought about how to respond tactfully, someone else stood up and supported the first speaker. A GH supporter shot back, "These are not appropriate comments. Of course children should be treated to improve their health."

But the opponents weren't silenced. They had lived and worked with the sometimes severe behavior problems of people with PWS. They worried about making them taller and stronger. What if the parents could no longer physically control their child? And wouldn't society be gentler towards a short, plump, disabled-looking person? Would making people with PWS look more normal just be setting them up for expectations they could not handle?

To Lee, not giving GH bordered on child neglect. But at some level he could understand why these professionals, who had been working with the syndrome for so long, were suspicious of these interlopers—these endocrinologists—coming in and saying, "Oh, we found a magical treatment for it."

There was no resolution at the conference, but the trend was in favor of GH. More parents—especially those of young children—went with their hopes over their fears. The following year, 2000, the drug maker Pharmacia got FDA approval to market its synthetic GH as a treatment for poor growth in children with PWS. Pharmacia asked Lee to head up a PWS board of consultants to spread the word on the benefits of GH. He brought in Janalee and Angulo. Use of GH in patients with PWS steadily increased.

It looked like the controversies were over. Then, out of Switzerland—the land where Prader-Willi syndrome was discovered—came a disturbing report.

Urs Eiholzer, a Swiss endocrinologist, was not a man who lacked confidence. He had broken away from Andrea Prader and the Kinderspital to form his own private clinic in Zurich, where he treated kids with PWS from Switzerland, Germany, and beyond. But he had always been nervous about prescribing GH injections for babies. It had been Prader, with his calm rationality, who had steadied and encouraged him. Prader told him that Eiholzer's own study showed that GH deficiency was innate, and that if he could show a GH deficiency, he should treat it. It didn't matter if the patient was six years old or six months old.

Then, disaster. Two of Eiholzer's young PWS patients died shortly after starting growth hormone therapy. One of them was just eight months old. Eiholzer was in shock. Had he caused the deaths by administering GH? He knew how devastating the loss of a child was. When Eiholzer was eleven, his younger brother had died in a car crash. There was no worse catastrophe.

He had a horrible fantasy: all of the more than ten very young children with PWS getting GH at his clinic would die, one by one. Every day he waited for the phone call announcing another dead child. The weeks went by, and the dreaded calls did not come. Eiholzer steadied himself and began to investigate the deaths. Both families, despite being deep in mourning, answered his questions patiently; one was Swiss and the other was Albanian.

It was never clear whether GH had contributed to the deaths of his patients. But Eiholzer came to appreciate that there was a subset of Prader-Willi patients with respiratory problems who were at greater risk of sudden death in general, and whose problems might conceivably be exacerbated by starting them on growth hormone. GH treatment was known to cause initial fluid retention, and might also cause tonsils to grow.

Eiholzer published his reports in 2002. A handful of similar incidents were subsequently reported. Janalee was now getting calls and emails from worried parents and care providers. She had put PWSA squarely behind GH treatment. Matt, now thirty years old, had recently gone back on GH, and had lost 30 pounds in three months from a combination of GH injections and a new exercise program. And there was so much evidence of the benefits of GH. Would they lose the one effective medical treatment they had?

Like Eiholzer, Janalee spent an anxious period, waiting for more reports of premature deaths that could be linked to GH. But no wave of deaths occurred. Pfizer, which had taken over Pharmacia, launched an investigation that produced results very similar to Eiholzer's. It wasn't clear that GH had contributed to the handful of sudden deaths, and if it had, it was because the patients had preexisting respiratory problems that might have been temporarily exacerbated by GH.

This was not so hard to fix. Pfizer put a new warning on its medication, telling physicians to watch for and treat upper airway obstructions and respiratory infections before starting GH treatment. Janalee reported all this in the July 2003 newsletter. She said there was reason for concern but not panic, and there was no recommendation to discontinue GH. Some countries stopped GH treatment for PWS because of the controversy. Some stopped it temporarily, then returned to it. The panic slowed, but in the end did not alter the trend toward use of growth hormone as the standard of care for Prader-Willi syndrome, at least in those countries that could afford it.

The entire GH experience showed how far PWSA had come. It had taken the lead in recognizing the value of GH treatment and in educating professionals. It had responded soberly to the sudden death controversy. The organization Gene had conceived and Shirley had midwifed was all grown up.

By the late 1990s, both geneticists and endocrinologists finally had something to offer parents. The former had a genetic test. The latter had growth hormone. But more was expected from the geneticists. They had performed a great feat in pinpointing the region of the human genome that was responsible for PWS. Surely this would be followed by more feats. Gene and Fausta felt buoyed up by the genetic discoveries, but would those discoveries lead to practical treatments for Curtis and all the others?

Twenty-Three

LESSONS OF GENETICS

The hope for future genetic breakthroughs kept bubbling up in the pages of *The Gathered View*. In the early and mid-1990s, more geneticists were drawn to studying the Prader-Willi region. Several genes were discovered in the PWS region. The imprinting center—the key stretch of DNA that was needed to allow PWS-region genes to be turned on and off in sperm and eggs—was discovered. Researchers found that mice had a region similar to the human Prader-Willi region, and they set about creating the mouse version of Prader-Willi syndrome. Other researchers searched for unique human patients with mutations in just one of the PWS-region genes, which they hoped would allow them to link the symptoms to specific genes.

In 1995 Suzanne Cassidy and Rob Nicholls made a bold claim in *The Gathered View*: "In the next few years those of us studying PWS will understand which gene(s) lead to hyperphagia [overeating] and obesity in PWS." Unfortunately for Gene and Fausta and Curtis and all the others, it was not to be. The mouse models were not as informative as researchers had hoped they would be. Many of the mice died in infancy. Those that survived did not develop overeating and obesity. And while a few unique human patients were found with mutations in specific PWS-region genes, the results did not provide clear answers. As of the writing of this book, the connection between the genes of the Prader-Willi region and the symptoms of Prader-Willi syndrome is still a mystery, and all the genetic knowledge has not led to any treatments.

Geneticists had more luck shedding light on why PWS keeps popping up in humans and what the risk factors are. The first mechanism to be understood was for the deletions. In the late 1990s, independent groups headed by Nicholls and Ledbetter discovered that at both ends of the common deletion—called the breakpoints—there was the same long segment of DNA. This large and unexpected "repeat" could occasionally cause DNA to misalign. In the busy sperm factories of human males, such a misalignment could cause a piece of DNA to be accidentally discarded on the factory floor.

The very structure of the human genome is the cause of the deletions. The risk factor for the deletions is simply being human. Every man with functioning testicles makes sperm that will cause Prader-Willi syndrome—thousands of them, every day.

We can estimate how many of the approximately hundred million sperm in the typical male ejaculate will cause PWS. Given that one in about fifteen thousand births is a child with PWS, and 70 percent of PWS cases are caused by a deletion in the sperm, simple math means that a typical ejaculation will contain about five thousand Prader-Willi sperm. It all comes down to which sperm reaches the egg. It's genetic roulette, and every couple having a child is playing it.

Geneticists were also quick to figure out the cause of the other major source of PWS cases. Only three years after the discovery that PWS can be caused by maternal UPD of chromosome 15, Suzanne Cassidy published a case study that clarified what was going on. A forty-three-year-old pregnant woman was concerned about birth defects. She had chorionic villus sampling at week eleven of gestation, which revealed that the cells of the placenta had trisomy 15, meaning three copies of chromosome 15, instead of the normal two.

If the fetus also had trisomy 15, then it was doomed; trisomy 15 is a lethal condition. But what sometimes happens is that early in the development of the fetus, one of the extra chromosome 15s is left behind during a cell division, creating a line of normal cells. These normal cells can then proliferate and outgrow the defective cells, leading to a normal fetus. This is called "trisomy rescue." And this is what happened in the case of the woman Cassidy wrote about. When amniocentesis was performed at week fifteen, the cells of the fetus looked normal: no more trisomy 15.

However, the baby girl was born with the symptoms of Prader-Willi syndrome, and genetic testing confirmed that she had maternal UPD of chromosome 15. If one of the extra maternal chromosome 15s had been left behind, the girl would have been normal. She would have ended up with one chromosome 15 from each of her parents. But instead, the chromosome 15 from her father was the one left behind.

This means that for every person with Prader-Willi syndrome caused by UPD, there are two other people who started with trisomy 15, but were restored to a normal genetic state when one of the extra maternal copies was discarded early in their fetal life. There are at least two thousand people with PWS caused by UPD in the United States. This means there are another four thousand who—quite unknown to them—almost got it.

Cassidy's paper established that UPD cases of Prader-Willi syndrome share a common mechanism with Down syndrome. Both have their root cause in an egg with an extra chromosome, except that in Down syndrome, it is chromosome 21, the smallest chromosome, and there is no trisomy rescue. In both syndromes, the chance of a defective egg increases with the age of the mother.

Some resourceful parents found ways to massage the cold facts of genetics into something warmer. One parent of a baby with PWS wrote in *The Gathered View* that they called their son their "limited edition" baby because, "after all, you only get a baby like him every 15,000!"

The mother of a child with PWS caused by UPD imagined her "special little egg" with an extra copy of her chromosome

15, waiting patiently "for its turn down the chute." "And when Mr. Sperm offered his 15th, my very independent egg said, 'no thanks, we're covered.'"

While parents were trying to make sense of why their children had Prader-Willi syndrome, another group—evolutionary theorists—were trying to understand why something as odd as imprinting had evolved. It seemed paradoxical. Why would mothers turn off certain genes in their eggs, and fathers turn off other genes in their sperm? Why would parents turn off perfectly good genes, depriving their offspring of a backup copy and making them vulnerable if anything happened to their one working gene?

The most widely accepted theory goes by the name of the "conflict theory." David Haig, an evolutionary biologist and geneticist at Harvard, argues that there is a subtle evolutionary conflict between the male and female interests in their offspring. Females value their babies equally. Males—whose babies might have to compete for their mother's attention and resources with half-siblings—care only about their own babies and not at all about some other male's babies. Therefore, males want to promote traits that make their babies more demanding of their mother's resources, while females prefer babies that are more manageable.

Haig emphasizes that males and females have a great deal in common in wishes for their offspring. Both sexes want their children to be robust and successful. Imprinting acts only at the margins. When females turn off certain genes in their eggs, they are relying on the sperm to provide a working copy of those genes. It's not that the female is trying to deprive her offspring of certain genes—she just doesn't want her babies to get a double dose. When a rare mishap occurs that eliminates the only working copy—as in Prader-Willi syndrome—the result is something neither parent intended.

Haig has written repeatedly about Prader-Willi syndrome. He has pointed out that the difficulties of newborns with PWS fit well with the conflict theory. Their poor suckling, weak or absent cries, and excessive sleepiness suggest that there are genes on the father's chromosome 15 that promote good suckling, a strong cry, and wakefulness. It's understandable that the mother turns off her copy of these genes. If she didn't, the baby would get a double dose and would be a real handful. It would be up all hours, sucking like a maniac and crying like a banshee.

PWS has been a gold mine not only for evolutionary theorists, but for medicine and science in general. Imprinting turns out to be important not just for PWS but for cancer, autoimmune diseases, and other disorders. In 2007 the editor-in-chief of the *American Journal of Medical Genetics* listed all the new concepts that PWS played a role in: microdeletions; imprinted genes; trisomy rescue; methylation tests for diagnosis; finding genes in the critical region; developing guidelines for health supervision; using multidisciplinary teams for treatment; establishment and growth of patient advocacy groups; and the collaboration of families, health care professionals and scientists in advancing knowledge.

As for Curtis and all the others with PWS, we can now say that their parents did nothing wrong to bring on the disorder.

PWS is not the result of poor nutrition or ingesting alcohol or drugs during pregnancy. It is not caused by men working with hazardous substances or otherwise damaging their sperm. The cause is a random error, either in a sperm or an egg. The risk factor is simply being human.

But despite all the new genetic understanding, there still was no simple fix for the behavior problems of people with PWS. Curtis, like many others with the syndrome, was still struggling. And there was worse to come.

Twenty-Four

CURTIS FINDS A NEW BOTTOM

The troubles at Laura Baker began when Bruce Jensen left. Jensen had led the Prader-Willi team, as Laura Baker expanded its Prader-Willi population from two to thirteen. Jensen was gaining recognition as a Prader-Willi expert—he gave talks at PWSA conferences. The staff at Laura Baker thought of themselves as a leading national center for Prader-Willi syndrome, second only to a PWS crisis facility in Pittsburgh.

In 1996 Jensen's third child was born. That fall the baby went in to day care, and Jensen bounced his first day care check. He thought, "I've got to get into a job that pays more, or I'm not going to be a middle class provider for my family." So he left Laura Baker to work at a glass factory.

After Jensen left, the board at Laura Baker hired a woman who, in Jensen's view, "just plain didn't like Prader-Willi people." She took actions to steer Laura Baker away from its focus on PWS. Curtis was placed in a small house with people with different developmental disabilities. He was expected to eat in the dining room with them and be satisfied with his small portion while they ate all they wanted to. The rules became more rigid and less adapted to the needs of the clients with PWS.

Curtis, now in his mid- to late twenties, was gaining weight and acting out more. To Gene and Fausta, the problem was not just the new leadership, but that some of the staff members—who were not well paid—lacked the education and know-how to deal with PWS clients. Curtis was increasingly unhappy. He came to feel that Laura Baker wasn't a very good place, that some of the staff were not very nice and would do or say mean things that made him angry. When Gene and Fausta tried to leave Laura Baker after visiting, Curtis would get in their car and insist on going home with them. They would have to get the staff to hold him back, screaming, while they drove away.

Kern and Ferron, at the Southern Cities Community Health Clinic, continued in their attempts to improve Curtis's situation with psychiatric care. Their main innovation was to substitute yet another SSRI, Celexa, for Luvox. But mainly their notes from the second half of the 1990s record the increasing problems Curtis was having.

In 1998 Laura Baker staff reported that Curtis had spoken of suicide during a couple of behavioral outbursts. Curtis told Kern that "lately I've been having a lot of stress." At his April

1999 visit, Curtis refused to consider Kern's suggestion that he go back on Buspar to help with his anxiety. Kern tried a new tack, talking to him about herbal remedies. He ended up taking valerian for its purported calming effects.

In fall 1999 Curtis refused to go to follow-up psychiatric appointments. In a December 1999 report, a Laura Baker staff member noted that Curtis had swung an ax around when agitated and had thrown objects about in a potentially dangerous manner. When he finally returned to the psychiatric clinic in late February 2000, he was adamant about wanting only "natural products" and to be off Celexa.

The day after his clinic visit Curtis refused to take Celexa any longer. Over the next week several staff members required treatment for injuries Curtis inflicted through bites and kicks. On March 9, 2000 it took five staffers to restrain a combative and threatening Curtis. The staff called 911, and an ambulance took Curtis to the Northfield Hospital emergency room, in restraints. Deana Antley went with him.

At the emergency room Curtis was placed on a seventy-two-hour hold. He fought off a nurse who was trying to take his blood pressure. He refused to take any medication. Gene and Fausta agreed to hospitalize him at Abbott Northwestern, a large teaching hospital in Minneapolis.

On arrival at Abbott Northwestern's mental health unit, Curtis swore at the staff and warned, "I'll kick your ass!" He needed restraints and the quiet room until he finally calmed down and rested. The next morning began with more yelling and threats from Curtis, concerning his breakfast tray. He calmed down and ate his breakfast, crying. Then he had his first meeting with the Abbott Northwestern psychiatrist who would oversee his care, James Knudson.

Knudson found Curtis alert and oriented, with no signs of psychotic thought. Knudson asked Curtis why he didn't want to take Celexa. Curtis said, "I have my reasons." He admitted having been aggressive toward the Laura Baker staff but did not express any regret. Knudson's impression was that Curtis had a mood disorder with aggressive/violent behavior toward others. He also noted that Curtis was stressed from conflict with the Laura Baker staff and his peers and from not liking where he was living.

He put Curtis back on Celexa and added Neurontin, a drug often used for anxiety and insomnia and as a mood stabilizer for bipolar disorder. Over the next few days Curtis acted somewhat manic—overly talkative, staying up late, scribbling all over the menu request form—so Knudson decided to drop the Celexa and increase the Neurontin.

Curtis stabilized: he lost his over-the-top aggression, and his baseline personality reemerged. He found many opportunities to get extra food. Once the staff caught him hanging around the breakfast cart—Curtis claimed he was organizing it. Another time he was found drinking a soda from another patient's room.

Curtis put off the nursing staff's attempts weigh him. "Later," he kept telling them. He also put off their attempts to get him to shower. Five days into the hospitalization, a nurse wrote, "body odor extreme." Finally on day six he consented to take a shower. He also finally consented to be weighed—he was at 172 pounds, well above his goal weight of 145, and nearly as heavy as when he'd first arrived at Laura Baker thirteen years earlier.

Socially, he had his strong and weak points. He was eager to make connections, participating in many of the groups at the hospital and speaking up. However, he spoke up a *lot*. Typical notes on Curtis: "Little sense of social appropriateness, interrupts constantly." "Needs repeated limits set on intrusive advice giving and disruptive commentary." "He was confronted on his use of humor at expense of others; he was not responsive to limits and then left the group."

Gene and Fausta played an important role in Curtis's recovery, warning Knudson about their son's bad reaction to Haldol, visiting Curtis repeatedly, and even bringing Curtis his cat. Knudson agreed to discharge Curtis back to Laura Baker on day seven of the hospitalization. Curtis was happy to be leaving the hospital. Then he got bad news: the Laura Baker staff heard that his weight was up and decided to reduce his daily calories to 1,200.

Crying and angry, Curtis refused to leave the hospital. There was a standoff that lasted several hours. Knudson had to be brought in. He managed to broker a deal: Curtis would remain on the 1,500 calorie diet for a day, then it would be reduced 100 calories per day until it reached 1,200 calories. And with that, the mental health unit at Abbott Northwestern bade farewell and Godspeed to Curtis Deterling.

But things were still going poorly at Laura Baker. Curtis continued to take the Neurontin, but that did not save him from what happened next. He began telling people at Laura Baker that Gene and Fausta were not his real parents and that his real family was the Dukes of Hazzard, from the TV show. After several days of that, he became terrified that the "hairy monster from Sesame Street" was coming to get him. On April 8, 2000 he barricaded himself in his room and stayed up the whole night. He was actually seeing the hairy monster. The next morning he decided to walk to California to join his real family.

Curtis managed to slip out of Laura Baker. A Laura Baker staff member who was driving around Northfield on errands spotted Curtis walking down the sidewalk. She asked him where he was going, and he told her, California. She managed to coax him into her car with the promise of a sugary drink, and she got him back to Laura Baker.

Once again, the staff called 911. The ambulance driver found Curtis sitting calmly in a chair. Curtis agreed to go back to Abbott Northwestern, saying he was going to show them that he was not crazy anymore. The driver noted that Curtis was speaking slowly and adding "E-O" to the end of every word.

Deana Antley stayed with Curtis as he waited for the ambulance. She could see his mind slipping away, as his ability to communicate deteriorated into "word salad" and nonsense words. She thought it was the worst thing she had ever seen.

Once back on the mental health unit at Abbott Northwestern, Curtis pulled himself together and did an intake interview. The nurse noted he was wearing an army fatigue jacket, with shorts and boots. He told her all about his plan to go to California to be with his real family, the Dukes of Hazzard. He told her he was at the hospital "to get checked out." Then he added, "I'm here to get freedom just like everyone else." And then, "Everyone who has ever treated me badly is going to jail."

She asked if he was married.

"Nope. But I'm gonna get one in just a little while."

She asked if he had children.

"Yes I do, I have four boys and four girls."

She asked what he expected to get out of this hospitalization.

"I just want to get the same respect."

She asked if he had any spiritual beliefs.

"No, not really. I believe in almost everything except for violence."

The nurse assessed him as delusional and having visual hallucinations, with a loose, rambling thought process. He looked sad and tired. Knudson was once again Curtis's in-hospital psychiatrist. He had a new impression of Curtis: schizoaffective disorder. Gene had told him that during his earlier psychotic episode, back in 1994, he had responded to Risperdal. Knudson decided to put Curtis on Risperdal, and to taper off the Neurontin in favor of Depakote (another medicine used to treat the manic phase of bipolar disorder).

Curtis showed little response to the new drugs, as shown in the nurses' notes from his first several days:

Day Two: Found in his room yelling at what he described as a "big hairy monster."

Day Three: Patient unable to follow staff directions to not yell, not run in halls and not roll around on the floor. Patient removed his clothes and attempted to enter female patient room naked.

Day Four: Curtis was observed taking his clothes off and was unable to give a reason why. This writer discovered Curtis' bathroom toilet to be overflowing with feces, with clothing in it. Made a slow dive into folded up ping pong table during Goal Setting group.

Day Five: Curtis pounded on his door, urinated on the floor of his room, and spoke of the hairy monster. But he did attend OT Clinic for 10 minutes and quietly sat down in Spirituality Group for a few minutes.

On day six, Knudson consulted with Kern, from the psychiatric clinic. Kern suggested a new antipsychotic, Zyprexa. Knudson talked it over with Gene, who was okay with a cautious trial. Curtis agreed, too. Knudson also prescribed Ativan, for anxiety. With these new medications, Curtis became conversational and pleasant, and stopped disrobing. On day nine, he told Knudson, "Hairy monster is not real at all."

Gene and Fausta visited Curtis several more times. Knudson came to rely on their insights into Curtis. Late in the hospital stay, Gene told Knudson that Curtis's behavior had deteriorated when he was off Celexa—so Knudson wrote a prescription for Celexa. The unit's social worker noted that

Curtis "has strong family support." On day eleven, Knudson discharged Curtis. The final nurse's note was: "Patient anxious and excited to be discharged to Laura Baker. Behavior in control, pleasant."

Gene and Fausta were relieved to have Curtis restored to sanity, but shaken by his consecutive breakdowns. It seemed like every promising start was fated to fizzle out. It was obvious that Laura Baker was no longer a good place for Curtis. But what other option was there?

Twenty-Five

The Last Stop

Marty McGraw knew when he was fourteen what he would do with his life. During his childhood in Litchfield, Minnesota, his mother had a friend who had a son—Jack—with Down syndrome. Jack and Marty were the same age, and by age fourteen Marty was looking after Jack. He didn't mind hanging out with Jack; he found him charming. Also, Marty had a sister, three years younger, with cystic fibrosis. Marty learned early that some people are given a tough hand to play and need help. By his early teens he knew he would spend his life caring for people with disabilities.

At the age of seventeen he joined the Army to get away from home and make some money for college. He was one of ten children. If he wanted to go to college, he would have to pay for it himself. After the Army he got educated, ending up with a degree in psychology and behavior management. Meanwhile, he worked in facilities for people with developmental disabilities. At one point he ran a home for seven people, on his own.

He first encountered Prader-Willi syndrome in 1977, when he was twenty-five years old. A woman named Doris Luhman started working as a cleaning woman at the home Marty was running. She was a teacher, with a degree in art. She'd taken the cleaning position because she had a three-year-old son, Matt, who had PWS, and she wanted to see what adult life looked like for people with disabilities.

Doris and Marty became friends. A few years later Doris asked Marty if he would take care of Matt and his sibling so she and her husband could get away for the weekend. When Marty and his wife arrived, Doris told them Matt had gotten into their beer and had drunk the better part of a six pack.

Marty hesitated.

Doris said, "Marty, I called the doctor. Just keep waking him up every once in a while, he's going to be fine. You know what? We are going on this trip! We haven't gotten away for seven years!" That was Marty's first time caring for someone with Prader-Willi syndrome. Matt made it through the weekend, and in fact Marty found him delightful, once the boy sobered up.

By 1992, after working under a series of difficult bosses, Marty started his own company. He named it AME, after his daughters, Anna, Molly, and Elizabeth. He opened a small home for three developmentally disabled people in Buffalo, Minnesota. Thanks to a national loosening of regulations in the 1980s, small homes for up to four developmentally disabled people could be opened in residential, suburban neighborhoods.

Doris Luhman began pestering Marty to open a small home for people with PWS. Matt was now a young adult. Doris had him on the waiting list for Oakwood, but she didn't see why the small home model couldn't work for people with PWS.

Marty said, "Well, Doris, it's not so easy. You need to…"

"What? What do I need, Marty?"

"You need three other people that have this syndrome, and have got funding. And you need a house."

She was back two months later. "I think I've got the three people, Marty. Where do you want the house?"

Doris had teamed up with Joan and Jim Gardner, whose son Larry had PWS. The Luhmans and the Gardners bought a house in Buffalo, and Marty opened his first PWS group home in November 1992.

Marty had spoken with the people running Oakwood, and they'd been dismissive of the idea that a small group home for PWS could work. They warned him that when a client with PWS was having a severe behavioral problem, Marty would need a lot of staff to restrain them. There wouldn't be enough staff at his little home. That didn't deter Marty. He figured that if he did a better job tending to his PWS clients, the need for physical restraints would be minimal. He created a structure that emphasized positive reinforcement—awarding chips randomly and intermittently for good behavior.

But Marty still had some things to learn about PWS. He initially had just one staff member at the PWS home—a top-notch employee. After six months the guy had had enough. He told Marty that the intensity of four clients with PWS was more than one live-in person could handle. While other developmentally disabled clients might let things slide, the PWS clients were sticklers. And they were smart, much smarter than the typical developmentally disabled client.

One time, Larry Gardner called Marty.

"Mr. McGraw, we were supposed to have graham crackers, that's what's on the menu. Instead we're having rice crackers."

"Oh Larry, that's not a big deal."

"You should know a little bit more about the syndrome if you are the owner and manager and ultimately responsible. If graham crackers are promised and rice crackers are given instead, well, that is very important to us."

Marty realized that he needed two staff members, and he also needed motivated and well-trained staff. When he opened his second PWS home, he told the parents, "We aren't going to pay them dirt wages, like other places." Instead of the going rate of nine dollars per hour, he paid his staff twelve dollars per hour.

Gene and Fausta heard about Marty's success in running small PWS group homes. In the late 1990s Gene would call Marty periodically when Curtis was in crisis, but Marty never had any openings. Finally, a slot opened up for Curtis in a new PWS group home.

At thirty years of age, on March 30, 2001, Curtis left Laura Baker and moved to Marty's new home in Underwood to join two women and a man, all with PWS. He was wearing a racing hat, jacket, and boots—all made of black leather. He was not in great shape. His weight had risen to 181, even higher than when he was first admitted to Laura Baker. His room was so full of stuff you couldn't really walk in it. At one point in his last year, a staff member became concerned that Curtis had some items in his closet that could be used as weapons. The staff member consoled himself with the thought that the room was so profoundly messy that Curtis's closet was essentially unreachable.

It took Gene and Fausta three trips to empty Curtis's room. He had more than a thousand matchbox cars, which they put in storage. They also found empty bags for loaves of bread, and an empty sugar canister.

After nearly fourteen years at Laura Baker, Curtis was getting a chance to start over. But he, and Gene and Fausta, were wary and scared. They'd all been through so much. Every promising start had ended in disappointment. This was the pattern for Curtis: not the happy, satisfying life Gene and Fausta had dreamed for him, but a downward spiral.

At the AME home in Underwood, Curtis continued the combative relationship he had grown accustomed to at Laura Baker. He liked to lie on his bed and watch TV. He didn't like to do chores or exercise or worry about his hygiene. As the AME staff tried to get Curtis to get with the program, he was making lots of calls to Gene and Fausta. "You won't believe what they are making me do. They really want me to take a shower."

Gene and Fausta tried to be protective of Curtis, and they sometimes took his word over the staff's. Four months in, Marty had reached a breaking point. He wrote a letter to Gene and Fausta, giving them notice that they would need to find another home unless they were able to cooperate 100 percent with his staff. Shortly after sending them the letter, he arranged a meeting at Underwood. Gene was off somewhere, but Fausta sat down with him.

Marty said, "So, Fausta, how have you been?"

"Since you wrote the letter, Marty, I've been very depressed."

"God, I'm so sorry."

Marty felt awful, but the letter got Gene and Fausta's attention. They didn't want Curtis kicked out of the home. They figured they had better shut up and not make waves, even though it seemed to them that a couple of staffers were too dogmatic.

As the AME staff and Curtis got to know each other, there was a bit of improvement. After two years at Underwood, Curtis had lost 20 pounds, and was having fewer disruptive behaviors at the home. But he was still resistant to exercise and hygiene, and he was dropped from his day program for stealing food and behavioral outbursts. He was also banned from the local library and the local YMCA.

In spring 2003, one of the two female housemates died from an infection after a transplant operation. It was another reminder of the seeming fragility of people with PWS. And would this sudden trauma cause Curtis to become despondent and have another mental breakdown? At least that fear was unfounded. Curtis's first response to the news was, "Well, who gets her movies?"

Marty moved Curtis and his male housemate to another PWS home, in Plymouth, where they joined two men already living there. The struggles continued. Curtis had difficulty completing his daily routines. He was refusing to do contract work at his new work site. He actively sought out food, stealing it from his housemates. One time he snuck a bag of kitchen garbage into his room and devoured anything remotely edible.

The AME staff decided to shake things up. They thought Curtis should see a new psychiatrist, one who specialized in developmental disabilities. Gene and Fausta agreed. Curtis first saw Ronald Hardrict in December 2004. Hardrict gradually tapered off Curtis's Depakote, increased his Celexa, and started him on a new drug, a mood stabilizer and atypical antipsychotic called Seroquel.

AME staff also decided to bring in a psychologist from the Minnesota Department of Human Services to review Curtis's functioning and recommend changes to his programming. The psychologist created a more detailed plan to track Curtis's behaviors. He also came up with a more tailored program for Curtis, focused on exercise, grooming, and daily chores, and reinforced by earning a variety of rewards including a trip to a pet store, eating a light meal at a fast food restaurant, going for a cup of coffee, visiting a car dealership, or seeing a movie. The AME staff reinforced the new program with a clear visual display that they posted in a common area.

The new medications and the new program, both started in spring 2005, had a positive effect. To one staff member, it felt like nearly a 180-degree change in Curtis's behavior. At a follow-up visit, Hardrict was pleased to see how much Curtis's behaviors had improved.

The AME staffers were also learning the best ways to work with Curtis. They learned not to take it personally when Curtis had an occasional outburst and became verbally abusive. And they learned not to talk at Curtis—telling him what he had done right or wrong—but rather to engage him, asking, "Curtis, do you understand why you did not earn that reward?" Gene and Fausta were pleased to see the improvement. But they remained clenched against the seemingly inevitable setback that would come and leave Curtis worse off than before.

The next year, 2006, was another year of growth for Curtis. The local YMCA agreed to let him back in, after banning him for four years. His completion of exercise, hygiene, and chores improved markedly. His behavior was calmer and more flexible.

AME staff decided to work on some of the finer points of his personality, including his tendencies when upset to call on a higher authority figure—trying to go over the heads of the staff—and to use racial slurs. They created a reward system and began tracking these incidents. They also addressed his problems with social interaction through "social stories." This involved discussion, role playing, and writing, to prepare Curtis for typical social situations when out in the community.

With Curtis's new, more flexible mindset, even social situations that he had not been prepared for could become learning experiences. In 2011, on an outing to a local Halloween event called the Trail of Terror, Curtis noticed a vendor selling incense. Curtis insisted—to the vendor's face—that the incense constituted voodoo paraphernalia. He also told the man's customers that they were buying voodoo supplies, that the scent was too strong, and that he just couldn't see why they were buying the stuff. Afterward the staff had a talk with Curtis about acceptable banter while in or near a person's place of business.

One day in 2012, Curtis went into the local bank. When he got up to the teller, he recognized her and said, "What was your name again?"

The woman smiled and said, "My name is Latrice."

"Oh yes, that's right. You have that weird name no one else has. Why would your parents give you such a weird name?"

Her smile a little thinner, the teller said, "My grandmother gave me that name."

"Why would your grandmother name you?"

The teller seemed to suppress a sigh. "Because sometimes it is hard for a person's parents to raise them."

The staff member with Curtis had been making increasingly frantic efforts to get Curtis to disengage from the conversation. Finally Curtis walked away. The staff member was Kevin Tobias, a burly former hockey player. He had joined AME just two weeks before Curtis arrived and had been in the same house as Curtis for over a decade.

After the bank incident, Kevin spoke with Curtis about how asking personal questions without permission is impolite. He also spoke with him about noticing visual cues when someone is frustrated or upset. Curtis admitted that he might have crossed a line and said he would not do it again.

Another difficulty that AME staff began focusing on was Curtis's tendency to pick at his skin, to the point of bleeding. Curtis lost a good job collating brochures for mailing because he was getting blood on the brochures. By 2012, the program coordinator at the house warned Curtis that if he didn't stop picking sores on his head, he would not be able to go out in public, other than for work, to medical facilities, to his bank, and with his family. The staff explained the health risks and gave Curtis literature. AME staff also created a system of positive rewards for not picking. With these explanations, threats, and incentives, Curtis finally made a conscious decision to stop picking himself on a regular basis.

With Curtis's behavior problems much diminished, the sweeter side of his personality could flourish. He used his free time to pick up trash on the side of 36th Avenue, near a high school. He told Kevin, "We owe it to Mother Earth to keep it clean. These teenagers need to stop littering." In winter, when he was done shoveling the driveway at the house, he would do the neighbor's driveway, too. Another of his favorite activities during free time was to go to the local humane society and give love to the cats and kittens.

Every year, Curtis enjoyed volunteering for the Minnesota PWS group's annual picnic. He told AME staff that he wanted everyone to have a good time, and he believed it was important to lend a helping hand. Every Christmas he bought gifts for others. He had found a new girlfriend, whom he saw several times a year. On Valentine's Day and on her birthday he became a model boyfriend, picking out gifts for her. Once he even sang her a song on his guitar that he had written for her, although the song turned out to be about God and the Earth. Curtis and his girlfriend made plans to marry, adopt four boys and four girls, and build a log cabin to live in.

Finally—finally—Gene and Fausta unclenched. The fear that each day would bring the news of some catastrophe faded away. The fear that Curtis would never be happy in his life, would never be a contributing member of his community, faded away.

Curtis came to see his AME house in Plymouth as his home. He had a stability there that he hadn't had since leaving his parents' home: Kevin, who was there from his first day at AME in 2001, became the head of the house. Curtis's sense of humor reemerged. He liked to call himself a lone wolf, so Kevin would teasingly call him "Tweety Bird."

"Oh yeah, what would you know, chicken-hearted Goat Boy," Curtis would shoot back, referencing the *Saturday Night Live* character. Then Kevin would bray like Goat Boy and Curtis would crack up. Kevin and Curtis and the other housemates liked to pick out some ridiculous movie to watch—often a horror film—and then laugh at it. Kevin said, "We're a laughing household."

Curtis was doing better at work, too. He was able to work in the community more than before. With his picking under control, he was back at the job collating brochures. His paychecks got a little bigger because he put in more of an effort.

When another AME client died suddenly and tragically, Curtis's response showed how far he had come. He was sad, and at the funeral, he went up to the grieving mother and said, "I'm sorry for your loss. He was a good guy."

At times Curtis's satisfaction with his life bubbled out of him. At Thanksgiving 2012 staff wrote: "Curtis talked about being thankful for such a great family. The rest of the conversation was how happy he is to have his new winter boots and to be living here at AME." The year before, at a Christmas party, Curtis stood up and toasted Marty.

In December 2012, Curtis went to a movie. After it was over, the lone staff member with him asked Curtis to sit on a bench and not leave it for just a minute so he could use the bathroom. When the staff member emerged one minute later, Curtis was over by the condiments. The staff member asked Curtis to empty his pockets and found twenty packets of sauces.

Postscript

I felt less alone after researching and writing this book. I enjoyed getting to know Gene and Fausta and Shirley, Marge and Sam and Janalee—the good people who founded and nourished PWSA. They are my spiritual parents. Shirley and Marge passed away after I interviewed them and before I finished this book, but at least I was able to thank them in person.

These ordinary and remarkable people also inspired me in my personal life. I'd been divorced from Naomi's mother since Naomi was a baby (the divorce was due to preexisting problems, not to Naomi having PWS). I wanted to get remarried, but I was not getting anywhere with the women I was dating. Seeing the abiding humor and love between the Neasons and between the Deterlings inspired me to work harder at finding my own Shirley, my own Fausta. I also drew inspiration from Sam, whose attachment to women is profound. Finally I met Luanne, and on November 15, 2014, we married. Our first child was born in January 2016.

I also felt less alone after learning the scientific and medical history of PWS. I felt comforted somehow that so many brilliant people had devoted chunks of their careers to puzzling out the mysteries of the rare syndrome. I was happy to learn that the genetics of PWS were fascinating and novel, and had larger implications. It made me feel that PWS is not some strange, pointless twig on the tree of humanity, but an integral part of the whole.

I wish I could have interviewed the two great pioneers of PWS, but they both passed away before Naomi was born. Hans Zellweger died first, in 1990, at the age of eighty. He took his own life, settling into his car with a bottle of his favorite wine and letting his garage fill with carbon monoxide. He feared that he was starting down the same path toward decrepitude and dependency that he had seen his older brother travel. Zellweger, who had shown so much compassion and understanding for people with PWS and their families, held himself to a harsher standard.

Andrea Prader died in 2001 at the age of eighty-one. Like Zellweger, his final years were not easy; when his wife Silvia died in 1995 after nearly five decades of marriage, he lost his zest and curiosity for science. But despite the sad ending, he had accomplished what he set out to do in life: make scientific discoveries. Besides discovering Prader-Willi syndrome, he discovered several inborn errors of metabolism and became a worldwide leader in the study of growth and puberty.

And finally, I felt less alone after getting to know Curtis. He cheerfully sat with me and answered my questions. He asked me questions about my children. I could see how much he enjoyed his group home and, especially, how much he enjoyed Kevin. Seeing all that inspired me to try to find a similarly warm, supportive environment for Naomi when she reaches adulthood.

Janalee Heinemann believes that if Hans Zellweger were alive today, he would take back his bleak assessment of the syndrome. He would agree that, as Janalee has written, "We Prader-Willi families have love, happiness, and a great deal of strengths." He would see that, with the right support, people with PWS can be the blessings that their parents first saw them as.

Thank you for reading. If you'd like to leave feedback or get more information, please visit the website for this book: www.pwsbook.pub.

Endnotes

General

I owe a debt to all the people who trusted enough in what I was doing to let me interview them or to share historical documents with me. I interviewed Susie Airhart, Moris Angulo, Deana Antley, Art Beaudet, Sam Beltran, Marilyn Bintz, Suzanne Cassidy, Curtis Deterling, Evan Deterling, Fausta Deterling, Gene Deterling, Sara Van Hall (nee Deterling), Tim Donlon, Urs Eiholzer, James Hanson, Christopher Hawkey, Janalee Heinemann, Bruce Jensen, David Ledbetter, Phillip Lee, Marty McGraw, Lota Mitchell, Shirley Neason, Rob Nicholls, John Opitz, Karen Orcutt, Peggy Pipes, Vic Riccardi, Ron Rosenfeld, Jeb Sawyer, Carolyn See, Sandy Singer, Rich Strobel, Kevin Tobias, Dan and Kathy Wett, Marge Wett, and Barbara Whitman.

The Deterlings gave me permission to obtain Curtis's educational and medical records, and Karen Orcutt graciously shared with me Curtis's public school file. David Ledbetter gave me a copy of an unpublished history he wrote about the discovery of the microdeletion on chromosome 15. The families of Marge Wett and Vanja Holm gave me copies of unpublished personal histories that Marge and Vanja wrote. Shirley Neason gave me a document she wrote about the circumstances of Daniel's death.

I'm grateful to those who were willing to read my draft and give me feedback, allowing me to correct errors: Suzanne

Cassidy, Gene and Fausta Deterling, Julie Doherty, Urs Eiholzer, Janalee Heinemann, David Ledbetter, Phillip Lee, Marty McGraw, and Rob Nicholls.

As a first-time author, I owe a special thanks to the people with publishing experience who helped me out: Ann Espuelas, a published author and friend who read early drafts and helped me find my direction; Milton Trachtenburg, a published author and parent of a child with PWS, who helped me understand how to write for a lay audience; Susan Leon, an editor who gave me valuable feedback and helped me figure out the title; and Susan Lang, who provided superb copyediting.

I want to thank Janalee Heinemann for coming up with the idea for the cover, and both her and PWSA (USA) for all the photos, except for the one of Curtis Deterling (wearing the jacket and tie, under the word "SYNDROME"), for which I thank Curtis and his parents. Incidentally, the woman in sunglasses to the right of the photo of Curtis is Janalee Heinemann, the boy in the upper left corner is Matt Heinemann, and the balding man in the upper right corner is Andrea Prader. Thank you also to Simon Avery, my talented book cover designer.

Some sources are cited repeatedly, so I have abbreviated them.

AP = Associated Press

IEP = individualized education program

Mgt of PWS, 1st Ed. = *Management of Prader-Willi Syndrome* (New York: Springer-Verlag, 1988) The first of three comprehensive chapter books on PWS published with PWSA (USA).

The two subsequent editions, in 1995 and 2006, are abbreviated *Mgt of PWS*, 2nd Ed., and *Mgt of PWS*, 3rd Ed.

MOBARR = Mount Olivet Behavioral Assessment Report and Recommendations

OSF = Orono School District file on Curtis

PWS = Prader-Willi Syndrome (Baltimore: University Park Press, 1981). The first significant book on the syndrome, edited by Vanja Holm and Peggy Pipes.

SCCHC = Southern Cities Community Health Clinic file on Curtis

TGV = The Gathered View. PWSA's every-other-month newsletter from July 1975 to the present.

Introduction

My memories, and some personal records, are the source for nearly the whole introduction. The two paragraph quotes from Hans Zellweger come from his foreword to *Mgt of PWS*, 1st Ed.

Chapter 1: Prader-Whatever

Gene and Fausta Deterling, along with their daughter, Sara, and son Evan, are the sources for most of this chapter. In Curtis's Orono School District file I found a letter dated October 5, 1973 from Bresnan that documented Curtis' dramatic weight gain by age two and a half. That letter is also the source for

Bresnan's apprehension about letting the Deterlings read the medical literature.

Chapter 2: A Fatal Syndrome

Biographical information on Hans Zellweger comes from Wiedemann, "Hans-Ulrich Zellweger (1909–1990)," *European Journal of Pediatrics* 150:451 (1991); from my interview with Phillip Lee (Zellweger was tall); from my interview with James Hanson, a protégé of Zellweger's (influenced by polio epidemic, interest in neuromuscular disorders); from *TGV,* July 2001, page 6, transcript of Prader's presentation to the 1984 PWSA conference (Zellweger was head of residents); from Sam Beltran, in the preface to *Mgt of PWS*, 1st Ed. (Zellweger started registry of floppy babies around 1946); and from Hans Zellweger, "Diagnosis and Therapy in the First Phase of Prader-Willi Syndrome," Chapter 5 in *Mgt of PWS*, 1st Ed. (he participated in efforts to unravel hypotonia in newborns). Zellweger's 1946 paper was published in *Helvetica Paediatrica Acta*, 1946, 5 (translated from German).

Biographical information on Andrea Prader comes from Milo Zachmann, "Andrea Prader 1919–2001," *Hormone Research* 56:205–207 (2002); from *TGV,* July 2001, page 6, transcript of Prader's presentation to the 1984 PWSA conference (Zellweger trained him in pediatrics); from Zellweger, "The HHHO or Prader-Willi Syndrome," *Birth Defects: Original Article Series*, V(2):15–17 (February 1969); and from my interview with Urs Eiholzer (Prader was from wealthy family, was ambitious to make scientific discoveries, but drove old car). Details of the discovery of PWS come from *TGV*, July 2001, page 6, transcript of Prader's presentation to the 1984 PWSA conference; from Zellweger's Chapter 5 in *PWS*, page 56 (crediting Prader's "astute clinical acumen" for the discovery of PWS); and from a translation of the original 1956 paper, with annotations by Urs Eiholzer, published as Appendix A to *Mgt of PWS*, 3rd Ed.

Prader, in his 1984 speech to PWSA, *TGV*, July 2001, page 6, said that he and his colleagues didn't know the cause or how to treat the syndrome. The death of Prader's first PWS patient, Albert, at twenty-eight, was reported in Laurance, "Hypotonia, Mental Retardation, Obesity, and Cryptoorchidism Associated with Dwarfism and Diabetes in Children," *Archives of Disease in Childhood* 42:126–139 (1967), page 138.

The two English doctors who thought PWS patients had a metabolic problem were Evans, "Hypogenital Dystrophy with Diabetic Tendency," *Guy's Hospital Reports* 113:207–222 (1964), page 221; and Dubowitz, "A Syndrome of Benign Congenital Hypotonia, Gross Obesity, Delayed Intellectual Development, Retarded Bone Age, and Unusual Facies," *Proceedings of the Royal Society of Medicine* 60:1006–1008 (October 1967), page 1008. Papers documenting PWS patients' excessive appetite include Hoefnagel, "Prader-Willi Syndrome," *Journal of Mental Deficiency Research* 11:1–11 (1967), page 8 (garbage cans, cattle feed); and Jancar, "Prader-Willi Syndrome," *Journal of Mental Deficiency Research* 15:20–29 (1971), page 23 (raw sausage).

Prader and Willi's report of their PWS patients' good natures is quoted in Forssman, "Prader-Willi Syndrome in Boy of Ten with Prediabetes," *Acta Paediatrica Scandinavica* 53:70–78 (January 1964), page 76. Zellweger reported on his fourteen PWS patients in "Syndrome of Hypotonia-Hypomentia-Hypogonadism-Obesity (HHHO) or Prader-Willi Syndrome," *The American Journal of Diseases of Children* 115:588–598 (May 1968); and reported their stubbornness and temper tantrums in "The HHHO or Prader-Willi Syndrome," *Birth Defects: Original Article Series* V(2):15–17 (February 1969). The 1972 review, further documenting behavior problems, is Hall and Smith, "Prader-Willi Syndrome," *The Journal of Pediatrics* 81(2):286–293 (August 1972).

Papers documenting other medical problems: Dunn, "The Prader-Labhart-Willi Syndrome: Review of the Literature and Report of Nine Cases," *Acta Paediatrica Scandinavica Supplement* 186 (1968), page 32 (eye problems, specifically, strabismus); Zellweger, "The HHHO or Prader-Willi Syndrome," *Birth Defects: Original Article Series* V(2):15–17 (February 1969), page 16 (speech defects); Spencer, "Prader-Willi Syndrome," *The Lancet* 2(7567):523–582 (September 7, 1968), page 571 (day-time sleepiness); Laurance, "Hypotonia, Mental Retardation, Obesity, and Cryptoorchidism Associated with Dwarfism and Diabetes in Children," *Archives of Disease in Childhood* 42:126–139 (1967), page 137 (scoliosis).

Papers documenting children given up to institutions: Jancar, "Prader-Willi Syndrome," *Journal of Mental Deficiency Research* 15:20–29 (1971), pages 22–23 (English eleven- and sixteen-year-olds); Forssman, "Prader-Willi Syndrome in Boy of Ten with Prediabetes," *Acta Paediatrica Scandinavica* 53:70–78 (January 1964) (Swedish baby boy); see also Sulzbacher, "Behavioral and Cognitive Disabilities in Prader-Willi Syndrome," Chapter 11 in *PWS*, page 157 (institutionalization for PWS was common in 1950s and early 1960s).

The Boston family struggling to keep their son with PWS alive is found in Hamilton, "Hypogonadotropinism in Prader-Willi Syndrome," *The American Journal of Medicine* 52:322–329 (March 1972), page 323. The risks of drastic intestinal surgery (jejunoileal bypass) are found in Soper, "Gastric Bypass for Morbid Obesity in Children and Adolescents," *Journal of Pediatric Surgery* 10(1):51–58 (February 1975), pages 55–56.

Chapter 3: A Drastic Diet

Bresnan referring the Deterlings to a dietitian is documented in two of his letters from Curtis's Orono school file, one dated October 5, 1973, and the other dated May 8, 1974.

Peggy Pipes's biographical details come from my interview with her, and from *TGV*, January 1976, page 3. Details on the Seattle clinic are in La Veck, "Federal Programs for the Developmentally Disabled," Chapter 2 in *PWS*, pages 17–18.

Vanja Holm's biographical details come from *TGV*, July 1977, page 8 (bio) and *TGV*, September 1977, page 8 (her focus on developmental disabilities); from See, "For Some Children Life Is One Endless Meal," *Today's Health*, January 1976, page 16 (Holm realizing she already had some PWS cases at her clinic); and from Fjermedal, "Passion for Food Causes Death," *Daily News-Miner*, Fairbanks, Alaska, August 20, 1975 (Holm saw her first patient with PWS five years previously).

Holm and Pipes's work with Russell and the other boys with PWS is documented in my interview with Peggy Pipes; in Pipes and Holm, "Weight Control of Children with Prader-Willi Syndrome," *Journal of the American Dietetic Association* 62:520–524 (May 1973); and in Holm and Pipes, "Food and Children with Prader-Willi Syndrome," *The American Journal of Diseases of Children* 130:1063–1067 (October 1976), page 1065 (chart showing that children with PWS needed on average just 60 percent of the calories of normal children).

Holm and Pipes's discoveries about their PWS patients' food behaviors and how unhelpful professionals could be, and their plan for complete environmental control, are found in Holm and Pipes, "Food and Children with Prader-Willi Syndrome," *The American Journal of Diseases of Children* 130:1063–1067 (October 1976). The help Peggy Pipes got from Shirley Neason and from Russell's mother is documented in my interview with Peggy Pipes. The textbook she dedicated to parents of children with PWS is Pipes, *Nutrition in Infancy and Childhood* (Mosby, 1977).

The wave of publicity in 1975 and later is documented in Vanja Holm, *LifeStory* (unpublished autobiography), Chapter 22 (the sequence of newspaper reports); in "U.W. Studies Food-Binge Illness," *The Seattle Times*, January 22, 1975, page A16; in Fjermedal, "Passion for Food Causes Death," *Daily News-Miner*, Fairbanks, Alaska, August 20, 1975 (AP article that was widely published); in AP, "Prader-Willi: Disorder Sees Victims Literally Eat to Death," *News Journal*, Mansfield, Ohio, August 10, 1975 (another version of same AP article); in Seligmann, "The Child Glutton," *Newsweek*, October 13, 1975, page 69; in See, "For Some Children Life Is One Endless Meal," *Today's Health*, January 1976; and in Bottel, "The Eating Disease," *Good Housekeeping*, May 1977, page 176. Details of how Carolyn See was given the *Today's Health* assignment are from my interview with her.

Chapter 4: Parents Band Together

Gene Deterling telling Bresnan he wanted to start an organization for PWS is documented in Bresnan's May 8, 1974 letter, found in Curtis's Orono School District file; and in my interviews with Gene. Curtis's weight loss once he started on Peggy Pipes's plan is documented by Gene in *TGV*, July 1975, page 3. Details of Gene contacting Peggy Pipes and getting in touch with Shirley Neason are from my interviews with Gene; in Gene's writing in *TGV*, July 1975, page 3; in Shirley Neason's account in *TGV*, May 1980, page 9; and in my interviews with Shirley. The source for Shirley's "tough lady" nickname is my interview with her.

Details of the Neason family's history come from my interview with Shirley and from Shirley Neason, "Our Experience with Prader-Willi Syndrome," *Home Life*, July 1978, page 42 (Baptist publication). Gene and Fausta, in my interviews with them, mentioned how talkative and curious Daniel Neason was.

Details on the first meeting between Gene, Shirley and Peggy Pipes come from my interview with Peggy Pipes. In my interview with Shirley Neason, she said Gene came up with the name "The Gathered View" for the newsletter. The initial name of the organization, Prader-Willi Syndrome Parents and Friends, is documented in the early newsletters, such as the first one, *TGV*, July 1975.

Chapter 5: Shirley Rising

On the growth of the organization: *TGV*, July 1978, page 1 (ten members received the first newsletter); *TGV*, July 1975, page 1 (Deterlings imagined a "nationwide organization"); *TGV*, January 1976, page 1 (fifty-one members); and *TGV*, November 1976, page 2 (180 members from thirty-three states and five countries).

On skin picking: *TGV*, January 1976, page 3 (Judith Gelb reported her daughter picked her skin, Shirley Neason responded that her son did, too); *TGV*, May and September 1976, page 6, and January 1977, page 5 (three other parents reported their children picked their skin); Holm, "The Diagnosis of Prader-Willi Syndrome," Chapter 3 in *PWS*, page 33 (skin picking found in 81 percent of cases of PWS).

Other issues discussed by parents in the newsletters: *TGV*, July 1976, page 5 (low calorie recipe); *TGV*, July 1976, page 6 (physical development, food for behavior modification); *TGV*, January 1977, page 6 (variability in food drive); *TGV*, May 1977, page 5 (gastric surgery); *TGV*, May 1977, page

6 (residential facilities); *TGV,* May 1976, page 5 (work programs); *TGV,* July 1977, pages 5–6 (starting a parents' group); *TGV,* November 1976, page 3 (bed-wetting).

Shirley's writing in the newsletter: *TGV,* January 1976, page 1 (saying she could use advice); *TGV,* January 1976, page 4, *TGV,* July 1976, page 5, *TGV,* September 1976, page 4 (book reviews); *TGV,* March 1976, page 5, *TGV,* January 1977, pages 2–3 (summarizing presentations by experts); *TGV,* September 1976, page 2, *TGV,* July 1977, page 3, *TGV,* September 1977, pages 4–6 (reporting on Margo Thornley); *TGV,* January 1976, page 3 (Daniel's skin picking); *TGV,* January 1977, pages 4–5 (advice for teachers on children with PWS).

Sources for the handbook: *TGV,* July 1975, page 1; *TGV,* July 1976, page 2 (it was initially a group project); my interview with Shirley (narrative of completing it on her own); Shirley Neason, *Prader-Willi Syndrome: A Handbook for Parents* (Long Lake, MN: Prader-Willi Syndrome Association, 1978), page 4 (how it was funded); *TGV,* November 1978, pages 9–10 (England, Australia); *TGV,* November 1978, page 11 (Spanish translation); *TGV,* January 1979, page 10 (370 of 500 copies sold within six months); *TGV,* September 1979, page 6 (sold out, reprinting); *TGV,* July 1978, page 1 ("superb accomplishment").

Sources for Daniel's life: my interview with Shirley Neason (all the information other than the following); *TGV,* January 1978, page 3 (spelling bee); *TGV,* November 1976, page 4 (new school for Daniel); *TGV,* January 1979, page 5 (getting outdoor-type locks for older siblings); *TGV,* September 1977, pages 4–7 (summer camp); *TGV,* January 1978, page 3 (Daniel's height and weight); *The Seattle Daily Times,* June 6, 1976 (algae, glue).

Chapter 6: Gene the Shepherd

On the early growth of PWSA: *TGV,* July 1975, page 1 (annual dues); *TGV,* July 1976, page 2 (all the information people wanted); *TGV,* January 1979, page 1 (desperate parents); *TGV,* May 1976, page 2 (recent articles on PWS); my interviews with Gene Deterling (working with Fausta); *TGV,* May 1976, page 2 (paying for secretarial assistance); *TGV,* September 1975, page 2 (memorial fund); *TGV,* March 1976, page 2 (more than four hundred dollars from memorial fund); *TGV,* May 1976, page 2 (Gene: memorial fund important help); *TGV,* July 1978, page 1 (ten members received the first newsletter); *TGV,* September 1976, page 1 (165 members).

On the Deterlings' move from Massachusetts to Minnesota, the main sources are my interviews with Gene and Fausta Deterling. Other sources are: *TGV,* July 1977, page 7 (Gene's new job title); *TGV,* July 1976, page 2 (Gene expecting to renew his focus on PWSA after the move).

Sources for Gene building up PWSA: *TGV,* July 1977, pages 1–2, 7–8 (the board, first board meeting in Seattle on May 27, 1977); *TGV,* July 1988, page 1 (Beltran: first organizational meeting was in Vanja Holm's Seattle office); my interviews with Gene Deterling (Sam Beltran was helpful in organizing board); http://www.pwsausa.org, About PWSA, Our History: 1990s (retrieved October 20, 2015) (named changed to PWSA (USA) in 1992); *TGV,* November 1977, page 1 (Gene encouraged local groups); *TGV,* March 1978, page 7 (report on Sacramento group); *TGV,* September 1978, page 4 (Australia group); *TGV,* May 1979, page 7 (Los Angeles group); *TGV,* September 1979, page 4 (St. Louis).

The story of the boy with the ruptured appendix was reported in *TGV,* May 1978, page 3, and the story of the girl with gallstones was reported in *TGV,* March 1980, page 10. Vanja Holm wrote about people with PWS having decreased sensitivity to pain from inner organs in Holm, "Medical Management of Prader-Willi Syndrome," Chapter 20 in *PWS,* page 266.

The parent who wrote that the newsletter was "our bridge off of a remote island in an often cold sea" was published in *TGV,* March 1980, page 4.

Chapter 7: Quirky Curtis

For Curtis in preschool through second grade, my information comes largely from the Orono School District's file on Curtis. For preschool: OSF, June 7, 1974 letter from Weinreb to Jackson (Curtis to attend Community Clinical Nursery School program in fall); OSF, February 28, 1975 Community Clinical Nursery School mid-year report; OSF, June 1, 1976 end-of-year report (CASE preschool class). For Curtis's personality at home, the sources are my interviews with Gene and Fausta Deterling, and with Curtis's big sister, Sara. Gene's optimistic statement around this time is in *TGV,* May 1976, page 2.

For Curtis's first year in kindergarten, the sources include my interviews with Gene Deterling (recounting meeting with the principal); OSF, memo to principal Ron Gilbert (school placement); OSF, notes by Joan Ball (case worker for Curtis); and OSF, November 2, 1976 psychological report (Marshall Watters reporting on Curtis). The wheelchair sign incident comes from my interviews with Gene Deterling. For Curtis's partial year in nursery school: OSF, report from Stubbs Bay Nursery and Child Development Center.

For Curtis's second year in kindergarten, the sources are OSF, Mrs. Fenholt's hints in working with Curtis (kindergarten teacher); OSF, notes by Joan Ball (case worker for Curtis); OSF, March 1, 1978 report of periodic review. For first grade: OSF, October 24, 1978 IEP; OSF, December 12, report on evaluation; OSF, May 22, 1979 report of periodic review. Gene's soaring statement was published in *TGV,* January 1979, page 1.

Chapter 8: Like Finding Family You Didn't Know You Had

Information about the second PWSA board meeting was published in *TGV,* May 1978, page 2. The initial plans for the first PWSA conference were published in *TGV,* July 1978, page 2.

Sources for details about Marge and Dick Wett: *TGV,* November 1978, page 7 (seven children, Dick Wett is an anesthesiologist, age of Lisa, daughter with PWS); my interview with Marge (Lisa second youngest, how Lisa was diagnosed, Holm made the diagnosis); *Charleston News and Courier* (AP article), March 8, 1981 (Dick Wett comment about more than three thousand syndromes).

Biographical details about Marge come from my interview with Marge (the welding class); my interview with her son, Dan Wett (Marge arm wrestling her sons); and mostly, Marge's unpublished autobiography (tomboy, getting into mischief, hauling carpet while pregnant, welding class).

For Marge getting involved in PWSA: *TGV,* November 1979, page 1 (Gene announcing first steps to start Minnesota parents' group); *TGV,* September 1978, page 3 (Gene reports first group picnic); my interview with Marge (involvement with PWSA started with Minnesota chapter, Gene asked for help with correspondence and contacts); my interviews with Gene and Fausta Deterling (being unable to keep up, Marge eager to help); Marge's unpublished autobiography (her past experience with Edina group); my interview with Marge (helping Gene and butting heads).

For the planning of the first PWSA conference: my interview with Marge (Gene organized the conference); *TGV,* January 1980, page 1 (Gene's concerns about stagnating membership growth); *TGV,* March 1979, page 1 (list of speakers and hopes that Prader would attend); *TGV,* January 1979, pages 2–3 (Gene not sure how many would come, asking members to send in form); *TGV,* March 1979, page 1 (more than seventy-five expected, venue is Leamington Hotel).

For the first PWSA conference: my interview with Marilyn Bintz; February 24, 2014 email to me from Vanja Holm's daughter, Ingrid (Vanja Holm, at her tallest, was four feet eleven);

my interview with Shirley Neason (behaviors of the PW kids, Zellweger interviewing kids); *TGV,* September 1979, page 1 (attendance was 165); my interviews with Gene Deterling (parents happy to be at a place where they didn't seem strange, him reassuring one flustered speaker, parents would have liked a simple cure); my interviews with Fausta Deterling (Zellweger was supportive and nice); *TGV,* September 1979, page 1 (glowing comments); *TGV,* September 1979, pages 1–2 (Gene and Fausta Deterling announced at conference they would resign, and Marge Wett appointed vice president).

Chapter 9: Puzzled Professionals

Most of my information on the first scientific conference comes from *PWS,* which itself was based on the presentations at the conference. The list of attendees is in *PWS,* page 12. James Hanson's biographical information comes from my interview with him. His presentation is found in Hanson, "A View of the Etiology and Pathogenesis of Prader-Willi Syndrome," Chapter 4 in *PWS.* Holm's zinc deficiency theory is found in "The Prader-Willi Syndrome: Directions in Future Research," Chapter 25 in *PWS,* pages 313–314. Holm's comparison of PWS to Down syndrome before the genetic cause of Down syndrome was discovered is in Holm, "The Diagnosis of Prader-Willi Syndrome," Chapter 3 in *PWS,* page 27. Harper, in *A Short History of Medical Genetics* (New York: Oxford University Press, 2008), page 147, wrote that 1956 was the year in which it was discovered that there are 46 human chromosomes; on pages 152–153 he wrote that the discovery of an extra chromosome in Down syndrome was published as early as 1958. In an AP article, "Prader-Willi: Disorder Sees Victims Literally Eat to Death," *News Journal*, Mansfield, Ohio, August 10, 1975, Holm is quoted as saying of PWS that "it's not chromosomal."

Zellweger wrote a book on genetics: *Chromosomes of Man* (London: Spastics International Medical Publications, 1977). His thoughts on possible genetic problems in PWS are found in Schneider and Zellweger, "Forme Fruste of the Prader-Willi Syndrome (HHHO) and Balanced D/E Translocation," *Helvetica Paediatrica Acta* 2:128–136 (1968), page 133 (chromosome abnormalities in 8 percent of PWS cases but scattered); and in Zellweger and Schneider, "Syndrome of Hypotonia-Hypomentia-Hypogonadism-Obesity (HHHO) or Prader-Willi Syndrome," *The American Journal of Diseases of Children* 115:588–598 (May 1968), page 597 (chromosomal disease does not cause PWS).

The presentations that tried to be of use to parents are: Sulzbacher, "Behavioral and Cognitive Disabilities in Prader-Willi Syndrome," Chapter 11 in *PWS*, page 151 (bite-sized rewards); Zellweger, "Diagnosis and Therapy in the First Phase of Prader-Willi Syndrome," Chapter 5 in *PWS*, page 66 (rules for feedings); Herrmann, "Implications of Prader-Willi Syndrome for the Individual and the Family," Chapter 18 in *PWS*, page 234 (list of problem behaviors); Nielsen and Sulzbacher, "Relaxation Training with Youngsters with Prader-Willi Syndrome," Chapter 17 in PWS; Pipes, "Nutritional Management of Children with Prader-Willi Syndrome," Chapter 7 in *PWS*, page 102 (importance of starting a low-calorie diet early).

Chapter 10: The Europeans Sniff Out a Clue

My interview with Christopher Hawkey provided most of the details for this chapter. The other major source is the paper he wrote: Hawkey and Smithies, "The Prader-Willi Syndrome with a 15/15 Translocation," *Journal of Medical Genetics* 13:152–163 (1976). Other sources: "Hypotonia and Obesity Syndrome," *British Medical Journal* 3(5567):694 (September 16, 1967) ("obscure [but] interesting syndrome"); Harper, *A Short History of Medical Genetics* (New York: Oxford University Press, 2008), page 167 (chromosomes were grouped A through G because distinction of individual chromosomes was often uncertain, D group consists of chromosomes 13 through 15); Hartwell, *Genetics: From Genes to Genomes*, 4th Ed. (New York: McGraw Hill, 2008), page 443 (description of translocations, most people with reciprocal translocations are normal because they have not lost or gained genetic material).

Sources for other European teams that found chromosome 15 abnormalities in patients with PWS: Fraccaro, Zuffardi, Buhler, and Jurik, "15/15 Translocation in Prader-Willi Syndrome," *Journal of Medical Genetics* 14:275–278 (1977) (Italy and Switzerland), page 275 ("little doubt" that chromosome 15 was involved in pathogenesis of PWS); Emberger, "Syndrome de Prader-Willi et Translocation 15-15," *Annales de Genetique* 20(4):297–300 (1977) (France), page 298 (improbable that this rare translocation would be repeatedly associated with PWS by chance); Zuffardi, Buhler, and Fraccaro, "Chromosome 15 and Prader-Willi Syndrome," *Clinical Genetics* 14:315–316

(1978) (PWS in male with 9/15 translocation); Kucerova, "The Prader-Willi Syndrome with a 15/3 Translocation," *Journal of Medical Genetics* 16:234–235 (1979).

That the researchers at the 1979 Seattle conference were dubious about the link between chromosome 15 and PWS: Sulzbacher, Holm, and Pipes, "The Prader-Willi Syndrome: Directions in Future Research," Chapter 25 in *PWS*, page 314 (chromosome 15 connection is only alluded to in a single sentence in a four-page chapter: "There are also reports of chromosomal abnormalities in the literature that further research could clarify."); "The Prader-Willi Syndrome: An Annotated Bibliography," in PWS, pages 317–338, page 322 (summarizing Fraccaro, Zuffardi, Buhler, and Jurik 1977 study: "This study shows that some P-W syndrome cases may be a result of a chromosome 15 abnormality, but that other cases clearly are not."), page 328 (summarizing Lucas, 1969: "A phenotypically normal woman who had 13 aborted pregnancies is presented. The woman was found to have a translocation involving chromosome pair number 15. The implications for P-W syndrome are that such translocations are found in some P-W persons and this case documents that an apparently normal woman can carry and transmit this error.").

Chapter 11: A Missing Piece

The major source for this chapter is a history that David Ledbetter wrote called "Discovery of the Chromosome 15 Deletion in Prader-Willi Syndrome" (unpublished). Other sources are my interviews with David Ledbetter, Vic Riccardi, Susie Airhart, and Rich Strobel, and a journal entry by Vic Riccardi dated May 12, 2005.

The opening quote, "Stupid endocrinologist. Everyone knows..." is from Ledbetter's history. Airhart, in my interview with her, agreed that it sounded like something Riccardi would have said. In my interview with Riccardi, he said he did not think he would have said it. However, his 2005 journal entry does say that he "questioned the wisdom of [chromosome studies on PWS patients as] heretofore [such studies] had been 'normal' or merely had 'coincidental' structural rearrangements."

Details of Ledbetter's life and career are from his history and my interview with him.

Details of Riccardi's life are from my interview with him.

Details of the sign-out conference are from Ledbetter's history mostly, with some confirmation from my interview with Strobel (he remembered Riccardi saying that David thought this patient had a chromosome abnormality but that he didn't agree) and from Riccardi's 2005 journal entry: "At sign-out rounds, David H. Ledbetter (then a graduate student working in my laboratory) questioned whether one of the two chromosome 15s was shorter."

My sources for Ledbetter going back to the lab after the sign-out conference and involving Airhart are Ledbetter's history, my interview with Airhart, and Riccardi's 2005 journal entry. Riccardi's high opinion of Ledbetter and Airhart as cytogeneticists comes from my interview with Riccardi.

That proximal 15q was a troublesome region, with a certain normal amount of "squishing," comes from my interview with Airhart. Riccardi setting up the blind test and Ledbetter passing the test come from Ledbetter's history, from Riccardi's journal entry, and from my interview with Airhart. Riccardi's reaction ("this was only one case") is from Ledbetter's history. Airhart, in my interview with her, quoted other people in the lab saying, "David, you're crazy…" and quoted Riccardi saying that Ledbetter had a bee in his bonnet about this chromosome 15 thing.

Airhart, in my interview with her, confirmed that she and Ledbetter later married. She talked about Ledbetter's passion to make a discovery, and the competitiveness between him and Riccardi.

For Ledbetter going into Riccardi's office and showing him articles on PWS and 15q, the source is my interview with Riccardi. For Riccardi calling Jack Crawford and arranging for a number of PWS and non-PWS samples to be sent, the sources are my interview with Riccardi and Ledbetter's history. For the resulting analysis, my sources are: Ledbetter's history; my interview with Riccardi (Airhart, Ledbetter and Strobel looked at the samples); my interview with Airhart (she, Ledbetter, and Strobel looked at the samples); and my interview with Strobel (he was the one who figured out why they had mistakenly thought they had seen a deletion in one of the normal controls). The paper they wrote described their efforts to explain the one person with PWS who did not seem to have a deletion: Ledbetter, Riccardi, Airhart, Strobel, Keenan, and

Crawford, "Deletions of Chromosome 15 as a Cause of the Prader-Willi Syndrome," *The New England Journal of Medicine* 304(6):325–329 (February 5, 1981).

The lab's earlier co-discovery of another microdeletion syndrome was reported in Francke, Holmes, Atkins, and Riccardi, "Aniridia-Wilms Tumor Association: Evidence for Specific Deletion of 11p13," *Cytogenetics and Cell Genetics* 24:185–192 (1979).

Sources for the journal article and the genetics society presentation are Ledbetter's history, my interview with Riccardi, my interview with Strobel (a lot of excitement and discussion after Ledbetter's presentation to the plenary session, and people calling him "Dr. Ledbetter"); and a November 2, 2015 email to me from David Ledbetter (Riccardi said program committee chair at the American Society of Human Genetics had suggested that the senior author should do the plenary session presentation).

Sources for Ledbetter taking over the lab: my interview with Riccardi (had falling out with top Baylor administrator Tom Caskey, which was an open secret, and then was removed and put on a smaller lab, and anyway neurofibromatosis was main interest); my interview with Ledbetter (Riccardi was way too independent to have a boss, he and Strobel and Airhart were basically running the lab, under nominal supervision of some faculty member, after Riccardi was removed, then Ledbetter got the job), and my interview with Airhart (neurofibromatosis was Riccardi's true research passion, and basically confirming the others' stories).

Source for Holm, Pipes, and Sulzbacher's excitement about the discovery of microdeletions: preface to *PWS* ("exciting findings"). The source for Ledbetter speculating that smaller deletions would eventually be found with better techniques is Ledbetter's history.

Chapter 12: Marge Rising

Sources for Marge's increased responsibilities: *TGV,* November 1979, page 6 (fundraising chair); *TGV,* January 1980, pages 1–2 (secretary, Wett home became the new headquarters for PWSA). Sources for Gene's final acts as head of PWSA: *TGV,* November 1979, pages 1–2 (group homes, committees); *TGV,* March 1980, pages 1–2 (urging support for new committees); *TGV,* May 1980, page 2 ("I am not terribly happy to announce this…"); *TGV,* July 1980, pages 1–2 (his peaceful good-bye). The new leadership positions were announced in *TGV,* July 1980, pages 1–2, including Gene's new role as secretary-treasurer and board member.

Sources for details on Shirley Neason: my interview with her (some communications problems, Gene would have liked to see more of the newsletters, she had article on PWS in adults published at the first PWSA conference, giving speech in Vancouver to parents); *TGV,* May 1980, page 9 (Shirley saying it made sense to have a local editor in Minneapolis, Shirley's farewell message); Neason, *Prader-Willi Syndrome: A Handbook for Parents* (Long Lake, MN: Prader-Willi Syndrome Association, 1978); Neason, "Our Experience with

Prader-Willi Syndrome," *Home Life* July 1978 (Baptist publication); *TGV,* March 1980, page 2 (Shirley is secretary of PW Association Northwest); *TGV,* July 1982, page 1 (Shirley came up with idea of committees); *TGV,* September 1979, page 7 (the specific committees); *TGV,* July 1980, page 2 (Shirley named vice president); *TGV,* September 1978, page 9 (Daniel Neason jogs with parents); *TGV,* January 1978, page 3 (Daniel won spelling bee, was in a regular fourth grade with normal kids, and weighed a normal amount for his height).

Sources for details about Gene and Fausta Deterling: *TGV,* September 1978, page 3 (Gene writing about picnic he arranged for members of local Minnesota group); my interview with Fausta (she worked with other women on opening Oakwood group home).

Chapter 13: Daniel and Shirley Move On

Sources for Gene urging people with PWS to write in: *TGV,* November 1978, page 1. For Daniel's letter to the newsletter: *TGV,* May 1979, page 3. For Daniel not considering himself handicapped: my interview with Shirley. For Russell and Daniel's restaurant scheme, and Shirley saying they planned for independence but people with PWS needed a lot of structure: MacDonald, "Victims of Rare Disease Dispel Myths," *The Seattle Times,* June 6, 1979. Daniel not being able to apply math: my interview with Shirley.

The source for Daniel's school experiences is my interview with Shirley. That Daniel was trim is documented in

MacDonald, "Victims of Rare Disease Dispel Myths," *The Seattle Times*, June 6, 1979.

The main source for the events around Daniel's death is my interview with Shirley, and a document she wrote, unpublished, called "Circumstances Surrounding [Daniel's] Death." Other sources: *TGV*, September 1980, page 5 (Shirley having told Gene months earlier to get a new editor); my interview with Fausta (getting a call from Shirley about the death); *TGV*, May 1980, page 1 (conference June 19–20 at Cape Cod); *TGV*, July 1980, page 2 (Shirley named vice president); *TGV*, July 1980, page 6 (Shirley made successful motion to add an education committee); *TGV*, September 1980, page 5 (Shirley's letter to the readers of *TGV* about Daniel's death); dedication to *PWS* (honoring Daniel Neason).

Chapter 14: Curtis Versus Elementary School

All the sources for this chapter come from the Orono School District's file on Curtis.

For third grade: October 26, 1979 conference with the Deterlings (behavior problem at home, too); February 24, 1981 periodic review (Curtis talking back, sometimes hitting); June 1, 1981 periodic review (Gilbert took over discipline, Curtis referred to District 287); http://www.district287.org/clientuploads/FACT_Sheets/District_287_Fact_Sheet%20Nov_21_2013.pdf (information on District 287).

For fourth grade until the District 287 evaluation: September 22, 1981 IEP (Corcoran hired as management aide); October 13, 1981 Corcoran log (Gilbert asked her to keep a record of problems in dealing with Curtis, Curtis misusing swing, Curtis calling Cooper a nincompoop); October 27, 1981 Corcoran log (eating from floor, eating goo); November 17, 1981 Corcoran log (ornery, carried thrashing from the room); November 18, 1981 Corcoran log (Curtis not in school, Fausta asking why he was favoring his arm); November 19, 1981 Corcoran log (super day); November 30, 1981 Corcoran log (Corcoran trying to teach math and Curtis mumbling she should be fired); December 1, 1981 Corcoran log (Corcoran taking pencil box, Curtis striking Corcoran); December 1, 1981 disciplinary referral (for striking Corcoran); December 2, 1981 Corcoran log (Curtis saying it was not bad to hit teachers).

For the events around the District 287 report: December 8, 1981 Johnson report (came with one other staffer, observed Curtis during music, did some math with Curtis, Johnson's observations and recommendations); December 8, 1981 Corcoran log (Corcoran amazed at Curtis's good behavior during District 287 visit, attempted confrontation over Speak and Spell); December 9, 1981 Corcoran log (Corcoran was extra nice the next day, felt mean for trying to trigger a tantrum the previous day for the benefit of District 287 observers); January 29, 1982 IEP update (behavior modification plan).

For the remainder of fourth grade, as staff implemented the new behavior modification plan: January 24, 1982 Corcoran log (Curtis very happy about rewards under new behavior plan); January 25–29, 1982 Corcoran logs (Curtis overall behaving well under new plan); January 27, 1982 Corcoran log (Curtis arguing about losing star for arguing); February 1, 1982 Corcoran log (Corcoran striking Curtis in the face); February 8, 1982 Corcoran log (Corcoran explaining new pink slip process); March 15 and 17, 1982 Corcoran logs (paying for pink slips by missing recess time); May 1982 periodic review (Curtis better behaved since implementation of behavior plan); various dates, Corcoran logs (popcorn parties).

For Curtis's personality: Corcoran's summary (notes on her year as management aide to Curtis); Cooper year-end report (Curtis often "responsive or friendly" in relationship with teacher); February 19 and 24, 1982 Corcoran logs (lunch with Jeanne Wong); March 9, 1982 Corcoran log (substitute teacher with Asian features); April 19, 1982 Corcoran log (field trip); Piers-Harris test on self-image; May 1982 report of emotional and behavioral disorders assessment; Corcoran's notes and tips for middle school.

Chapter 15: A Home of Their Own

My main source for details about Lisa Wett while she was living with her family was Marge Wett. Other sources: AP article in *The News and Courier*, March 8, 1981 (mainstreaming Lisa in junior high was a disaster, Marge burned out two years ago); my interview with Dan and Kathy Wett (Lisa badgering Marge for food, sneaking it at night, cookies under the pillow, bungie cord on door; youngest Wett child, Andrew, might have missed out some); AP article, "Young

Compulsive Eaters Find Help at Prader-Willi Homes," *Reading Eagle*, May 30, 1984 (strain of Lisa too much for family, Marge feeling guilty).

Sources for Oakwood: *TGV*, November 1980, page 2 (waiting for final approval, capacity of fifteen); AP article in *The News and Courier*, March 8, 1981 (people asking Marge how she and Dick can put their daughter in a home); Covert, "For Prader-Willi Victims, Appetite Is Illness," *Star Tribune* (date unknown, have copy in my file; Marge saying that Lisa would happily go with neighbors if offered more food); *TGV*, March 1981, pages 4–7 (Marge on group homes and programs for people with PWS); *TGV*, November 1981, page 6 (Oakwood opening); AP article, "Young Compulsive Eaters Find Help at Prader-Willi Homes," *Reading Eagle*, May 30, 1984 (Lisa at Oakwood); my interview with Marge (Lisa visiting her from Oakwood).

Sources for Dorothy Thompson and Marge Wett working on more group homes: Dorothy G. Thompson obituary, *Star Tribune*, July 4, 2010 (was director of residential facility); *TGV*, September 1989, page 3 (two people with PWS taking up 90 percent of staff's time); *TGV*, July 7, 2010, pages 14–15 (Thompson helped open Oakwood); *TGV*, November 1987, page 5 (Thompson instrumental in getting homes opened, twenty-one group homes now versus one in 1979); *TGV*, March 1988, page 9 (Thompson traveling to groups opening homes); my interview with Marge Wett (Thompson and Marge traveled a lot, helping with state chapters and group homes); *TGV*, January 1984, page 1 (now 1,350 members in PWSA).

Sources for Andrea Prader: *TGV*, March 1984 (annual conference to be held in June, in Minneapolis); Zachmann, "Andrea Prader 1919–2001," *Hormone Research* 56:205–207 (2002) (he was "internationally famous"); my interview with Urs Eiholzer (Italians bringing children with PWS to kneel before Prader); *TGV*, September 1981, page 7 (parent reports on meeting Prader); my interview with James Hanson (Prader coming to Iowa and eating steak); *TGV*, July 2001, page 6 (Janalee Heinemann recounting Prader's visit to Oakwood; transcript of his presentation to the 1984 PWSA conference); my interview with Marge Wett (Prader overwhelmed by PWSA); *TGV*, July 1984, page 1 (attendance at conference more than four hundred).

Chapter 16: Curtis Moves Out

For Curtis's middle school experiences, all the sources are in the Orono School District file on Curtis: December 15, 1982 conference report (Martha Brown is management aide, only two time-outs needed, parents "very satisfied with middle school progress"); December 15, 1982 IEP (three lofty behavior goals for Curtis); November 21, 1983 annual review (following directions 40 percent of the time, being polite and considerate 50 percent); November 6, 1984 IEP (goal that Curtis follow directions without arguing 60 percent of the time); May 22, 1985 periodic review (following directions without arguing 50 percent of the time); May 2, 1984 incident (Curtis attacked Brown over cookies); August 31, 1984 report (Curtis in mainstream science in sixth grade but to change to direct service with Shay for seventh grade); February 13, 1986 report (Curtis in mainstream homeroom, art/computer, music, study hall); February 7, 1984 report (Brown to handle knife in art class); May 1, 1986 report (Curtis talking on and on and peers not liking it); April 17, 1984 conference to discuss Curtis's behavior ("I can't hear you when you're shouting"); March 12, 1987 (Gene saying "Curtis can't be pushed"); January 7, 1986 phone conference with Fausta (Curtis refusing to work, Fausta saying he would be disappointed not to go to neighborhood high school); May 23, 1986 periodic review (accepted by educable mentally retarded program); undated (Curtis referred to emotional/behavior disorders educable mentally retarded classroom at St. Louis Park High School, classroom structured for his specific behavior problems); March 2, 1987 note of call to Fausta (Curtis at impasse with teacher).

For Curtis's acting out at home: my interviews with Gene and Fausta Deterling and Curtis's sister, Sara (shoplifting food, Sara finding bunch of candy wrappers under the couch, Curtis trying to order six large pizzas); Lanpher, "Deadly Hunger," *St. Paul Pioneer Press* April 7, 1991, page 1F; my interview with Gene (one night Gene and Fausta woke to hear Curtis trying to get into locked food cabinets with a saw and realized they had to find another home for him).

Sources for finding a facility for Curtis: my interview with Sandy Singer (Curtis knew Oakwood but wouldn't move in, saying he wasn't like those people); www.laurabaker.org (retrieved April 25, 2014) (serves those with developmental disabilities and also mental illness); interview with Gene and

Fausta Deterling (Dorothy Thompson found Laura Baker for Curtis, who was opposed to going until Gene offered to get him a large trunk); Laura Baker file on Curtis (admitted June 7, 1987, weight and height noted).

Source for up to 50 percent of people with PWS seeming not to have the 15q deletion: Ledbetter, Mascarello, Riccardi, "Chromosome 15 Abnormalities and the Prader-Willi Syndrome: A Follow-Up Report of 40 Cases," *American Journal of Human Genetics* 34:278–285 (1982).

Chapter 17: The Great Genetics Mystery

For the Sherlock Holmes quote, see Doyle, *The Sign of Four* (London: Spencer Blackett, 1890), page 93.

Prader-Willi researchers who believed that all patients with classic PWS had the deletion: Mattei, "Prader-Willi Syndrome and Chromosome 15," *Human Genetics* 64:356–362 (1983), page 361; Niikawa, "Clinical and Cytogenetic Studies Of The Prader-Willi Syndrome: Evidence of Phenotype-Karyotype Correlation," *Human Genetics* 69:22–27 (1985), page 25; *TGV,* July 2001, page 11 (Prader, in speech at 1984 PWSA conference: "The great majority, or possibly all of the typical patients have a partial defect of the chromosome 15").

For Suzanne Cassidy, biographical details come from my interview with her. Other sources: Cassidy, "Prader-Willi Syndrome," *Current Problems in Pediatric and Adolescent Health Care* 14(1):155 (January 1984) (her monograph); Labidi and Cassidy, "A Blind Prometaphase Study of Prader-Willi Syndrome: Frequency and Consistency in Interpretation of

Del 15q," *American Journal of Human Genetics* 39:452–460 (1986) (70 percent had the deletion).

For Zellweger's red herring theory: *TGV,* September 1984, page 10 (doubtful whether 15q deletion causes PWS); Zellweger, "Prader-Willi Syndrome with Rare Chromosome Anomaly," *American Journal of Medical Genetics* (PWS Conference Abstracts) 28:915–924 (1987), page 915 (same); Zellweger, "Genetic Heterogeneity of the Prader-Willi Syndrome," *American Journal of Medical Genetics* (PWS Conference Abstracts) 28:915–924 (1987), page 920 (same). That the opposite view made a lot more sense, see Ledbetter and Mascarello, letter to the editor in *TGV.* May 1981, page 5.

For the theory that there would be smaller deletions in chromosome 15q that also caused PWS: Ledbetter and Mascarello, letter to the editor in *TGV,* May 1981, page 5 (deletions may be too small to find with current techniques); my interview with Suzanne Cassidy (we thought all patients with PWS would have the deletions but smaller than could be seen at the time); my interview with Ledbetter (fluorescence in situ hybridization [FISH] is much better technique than high-resolution chromosome analysis; his lab used FISH to find smaller deletions in Miller-Dieker syndrome).

Most of the biographical details for Tim Donlon come from my interview with him. Other sources: Latt, "The Use of Chromosome Flow Sorting and Cloning to Study Amplified DNA Sequences," in *Gene Amplification,* edited by Schimke (Cold Spring Harbor Laboratory: CSH, 1982), pages 283–284 (lasers and fluorescence); Donlon, "Isolation of Molecular

Probes Associated with the Chromosome 15 Instability in the Prader-Willi Syndrome," *Proceedings of the National Academy of Sciences* 83:4408–4412 (June 1986), pages 4410–4411 (15q probes deleted in one patient with PWS but not the other); Donlon, "Similar Molecular Deletions on Chromosome 15q11.2 Are Encountered in Both the Prader-Willi and Angelman Syndromes," *Human Genetics* 80:322–328 (1988), page 324 (five patients with PWS had the same deletion, and a sixth had no molecularly detectable deletion).

For Merlin Butler, the sources are: Butler, "Parental Origin of Chromosome 15 Deletion in Prader-Willi Syndrome," *The Lancet* 1(8336):1285–1286 (June 4, 1983); Hall, "Genomic Imprinting: Review and Relevance to Human Diseases," *American Journal of Human Genetics* 46:857–873 (1990), page 857 (genomic imprinting is quite contrary to basic Mendelian tenet that parental source does not affect gene expression).

For Ellen Magenis, the sources are: Kaplan, "Clinical Heterogeneity Associated with Deletions in the Long Arm of Chromosome 15: Report of 3 New Cases and Their Possible Genetic Significance," *American Journal of Medical Genetics* 28:45–53 (1987) (from Latt's lab, one of the three cases had Angelman syndrome); my interview with Tim Donlon (he told Magenis about the Angelman patient with the 15q deletion); my interview with Suzanne Cassidy (Ellen Magenis was an excellent "old-timey" cytogeneticist); Magenis, "Is Angelman Syndrome an Alternate Result of del(15)(q11q13)?," *American Journal of Medical Genetics* 28:829–838 (1987); Donlon, "Similar Molecular Deletions on Chromosome 15q11.2

Are Encountered in Both the Prader-Willi and Angelman Syndromes," *Human Genetics* 80:322–328 (1988).

For Art Beaudet, the sources are: Spence and Beaudet, "Uniparental Disomy as a Mechanism for Human Genetic Disease," *American Journal of Human Genetics* 42:217–226 (1988), page 217 (gene for cystic fibrosis mapped to long arm of chromosome 7 in 1985, girl inherited two chromosome 7s from her mother), page 224 ("A third pathological mechanism might involve requirements for chromosomal contributions from both parents"); my interview with Art Beaudet (finding out about the girl with CF and short stature, saying he and Ledbetter were stupid not to have realized that UPD could explain PWS cases without deletions); Engel, "A New Genetic Concept: Uniparental Disomy and Its Potential Effect, Isodisomy," *American Journal of Medical Genetics* 6:137–143 (1980); McGrath, "Completion of Mouse Embryogenesis Requires Both the Maternal and Paternal Genomes," *Cell* 37:179–183 (1984); Surani, "Development of Reconstituted Mouse Eggs Suggests Imprinting of the Genome during Gametogenesis," *Nature* 308:548–550 (April 5, 1984); my interview with Ledbetter ("Art and I kick ourselves in the butt all the time for not putting this together with Prader Willi syndrome.")

Chapter 18: One Puzzle Solved

For Rob Nicholls's biographical details, my main source is an interview he did with the Oral History and Archive Project for the Pew Scholars Program in the Biomedical Sciences in 1997.

Other details come from my interview with Rob Nicholls (his sister's illness gave him an interest in science and medicine; to work on human genetic disease he needed to go to England or the United States; Oxford accepted him; he hadn't heard of PWS but was immediately intrigued, as it was the reverse of his sister's problem).

For Nicholls's discoveries at Sam Latt's lab: Knoll, Nicholls and Magenis, "Angelman and Prader-Willi Syndromes Share a Common Chromosome 15 Deletion but Differ in Parental Origin of the Deletion," *American Journal of Medical Genetics* 32:285–290 (1989); Nicholls's Pew interview (Nicholls worried that someone else would figure out that UPD and imprinting explained PWS genetics and present it first, trouble proving UPD and serendipity of high voltage); Cram, "In Memoriam: Samuel A. Latt (1938–1988)," *Cytometry* 10:1–2 (1989); my interview with Nicholls (Howard Hughes Medical Institute, serendipity of high voltage); Nicholls, "Genetic Imprinting Suggested by Maternal Heterodisomy in Non-Deletion Prader-Willi Syndrome," *Nature* 342:281–285 (November 16, 1989); my interview with Ledbetter ("Art and I kick ourselves in the butt all the time for not putting this together with Prader-Willi syndrome."); September 19, 2012 email from John Opitz to John Storr; Zachmann, "Andrea Prader 1919–2001," *Hormone Research* 56:205–207 (2002) (Prader born December 23, 1919); Prader, preface to *Prader-Willi Syndrome and Other Chromosome 15q Deletion Disorders* (New York: Spring-Verlag 1992); April 29, 2014 email from Rob Nicholls to John Storr (details of position at University of Florida).

Chapter 19: Tentative Steps

My sources for Curtis's transition to Laura Baker and his early days there: my interviews with Gene and Fausta Deterling (trip to Alaska, no phone calls or visits for two weeks, Fausta's feelings, writing a letter to Curtis); www.laurabaker.org (retrieved September 23, 2014) (residential school was founded in 1897); my interview with Deana Antley (Laura Baker had seventy-six clients when Curtis moved in, Curtis was one of the early people with PWS at Laura Baker, older clients often forgotten by families, Gene and Fausta visited Curtis and took him home often); my interview with Bruce Jensen (Curtis very bonded with parents and went home with them at least twice a month); OSF, July 2, 1987 Laura Baker thirty-day review (Curtis argumentative and emotional, weighed 175); OSF, November 19, 1987 Laura Baker report (weight now 146, now taking regular showers, generally in calm state with few instances of physical aggression).

For Curtis's life at Laura Baker, after the first few months: my interview with Bruce Jensen (details of Jensen's life and experiences with Curtis); my interview with Deana Antley (Curtis chatting with her); OSF, April 10, 1988 report by Ann Strawn, management aide (Curtis showed extroverted personality, more tolerant of teasing); OSF, April 10, 1988 progress report (Curtis chatting with other boys about cars, wanting to be a pediatrician, falling asleep in English class and frustrated with Logo, not keeping up academically); OSF, October 16, 1988 Laura Baker report on use of floor restraint when Curtis would not change sheets); OSF, June 9, 1989 report from Northfield special education department (Curtis misbehaving and seeming to enjoy it); OSF, September 5, 1989 goals and objectives report (Curtis to attend graduation ceremony and receive certificate).

For Curtis's work experiences, the sources are from the Orono School District file on Curtis: May 25, 1990 meeting on Curtis's future (discussing workshop or supportive employment); June 30, 1990 letter from Root to Deterlings (enrolling Curtis at Dakota County Technical Center and setting up assessment); August 26, 1991 summary of Curtis's first year after high school (maintenance work); fall 1991 work/behavior contract; November 19, 1990 IEP update meeting (salvaging Curtis's job at the ice arena); November 2, 1990 IEP (Curtis to attend the technical center for career exploration, and to attend classes); March 10, 1992 vocational evaluation report (including Garley's office).

For Curtis's quality of life: my interview with Antley (quality of life was good before onset of psychiatric problems, various community activities Curtis and other Laura Baker clients attended, Curtis was a hoarder); MOBARR, September 24, 1994 (things Curtis enjoyed, including at his parents' house, and his collections); en.wikipedia.org/wiki/Northfield,_Minnesota#Defeat_of_Jesse_James_Days (retrieved December 28, 2014) (held annually in early September).

Chapter 20: A Drug for PWS Behaviors?

For Curtis on Prozac, my sources are: en.wikipedia.org/w/index. php?title=Fluoxetine&oldid=686676229 (retrieved October 20,

2015) (Prozac is an antidepressant in the SSRI class); *TGV,* March 1991, page 8 (Prozac typically takes two to four weeks before seeing any positive effect, Prozac and weight loss); Dech, "The Use of Fluoxetine in an Adolescent with Prader-Willi Syndrome," *Journal of the American Academy of Child and Adolescent Psychiatry* 30(2):298–302 (March 1991); my interview with Gene and Fausta Deterling (they heard about Prozac at a PWSA conference and convinced his doctor to try it, Curtis did not do well on 60 mg); OSF, December 18, 1991 Laura Baker team meeting summary (Prozac started February 21, 1991 at 20 mg/day, Jensen saw positive effects, by fall Curtis was back to baseline of misbehavior and increase to 40 mg didn't help); SCCHC, January 20, 1993 Ferron report (Curtis's history with Prozac, on 60 mg he became more agitated, Prozac dosage was lowered and Buspar added).

For Curtis's treatment by Ferron and Kern, up to his breakdown, all my sources are from SCCHC, other than one download from the web: June 22, 1993 report (first time Kern was involved); August 31, 1993 report (trying Zoloft); en.wikipedia.org/w/index.php?title=Sertraline&ol did=686007399 (retrieved October 20, 2015) (Zoloft is an antidepressant in the SSRI class); September 14, 1993 report (improvement on Zoloft at 50 mg); October 19, 1993 report (more verbal outbursts and very talkative, increased Zoloft to 100 mg); December 16, 1993 report (problems on 100 mg of Zoloft); April 21, 1994 (Zoloft discontinued as not consistently useful); May 31, 1994 (Ferron to discuss other medications with parents, going back on Zoloft); July 14, 1994 (Curtis doing well back on Zoloft, looking forward to PWSA conference).

For Curtis's experiences at the 1994 PWSA conference and immediately afterward: http://www.pwsausa.org, About PWSA, Our History: 1990s (retrieved October 20, 2015) (1994 conference was in Atlanta); SCCHC, August 1, 1994 report (Dr. Chang: Curtis was looking forward to PWSA conference, was shocked by girlfriend's weight gain and friend's death, became sad and apathetic, Gene changed Curtis's medications); MOBARR, September 24, 1994 (Curtis excited about upcoming PWSA conference, was quite shocked at Page's weight gain, refused to attend banquet and dance, Curtis's difficulties with family on Cape Cod); my interview with Marilyn Bintz (details on Page's life); my interview with Gene and Fausta Deterling (Curtis on Cape Cod saying he wanted to bite Fausta, trip to the emergency room, Haldol made Curtis zombie-like); www.livestrong.com/article/177215-alleviating-side-effects-of-haldol (retrieved October 20, 2015) (Benadryl is used to counteract side effects of Haldol).

For Curtis's two initial hospitalizations after returning home, the sources are: my interview with Gene and Fausta Deterling (first trip to hospital, Evan outraged when Curtis was put in isolation during the second hospitalization; Laura Baker behavioral analyst Jensen recommended Mount Olivet); SCCHC, August 1, 1994 report (Curtis acting disoriented and guilty, hospitalization recommended); MOBARR (Chang saw Curtis August 1, decision made to hospitalize at Fairview Riverside, no organic cause found at Fairview, medications given, Curtis slept through two nights, discharged August 8, returned to Laura Baker August 12, problems on return to

Laura Baker, problems observed by EPIC staff); interview with Bruce Jensen (Curtis covered in feces, Jensen looked for a place to help Curtis and found Mount Olivet).

For Curtis's time at Mount Olivet, the sources are: www.mtolivetrollingacres.org/programs_services/crisis_transition_respite.html (retrieved December 12, 2014) (description of special services program); MOBARR (Curtis admitted August 17, 1994 and left for Laura Baker October 7, 1994, examples of his perseverative speech, chart of target behaviors by week, drugs given to counteract side effects of other drugs, side effects of drugs received at emergency room on Cape Cod, analysis of what led to his problems); my interview with Gene and Fausta Deterling (Fausta thought Mount Olivet was a great place and he was a lot better when he left it).

For Curtis's experiences after leaving Mount Olivet, my sources are: my interview with Bruce Jensen (Curtis was flatter after the psychotic break, lost his belly laugh); SCCHC, November 1, 1994 report (parents felt Risperdal sedated Curtis); SCCHC, December 6, 1994 report (parents wanted to minimize Risperdal); SCCHC, January 4, 1995 (parents wanted Risperdal discontinued, Kern and Ferron agreed); en.wikipedia.org/w/index.php?title=Fluvoxamine &oldid=675654151 (retrieved October 20, 2015) (Luvox is an SSRI); SCCHC, February 22, 1995 report (Curtis had a hard time off Risperdal but was opposed to restarting it, Kern suggested Luvox); SCCHC, March 15, 1995 report (not doing great, Luvox increased to 50 mg); SCCHC, April 18, 1995 (doing much better, medications continued as before); SCCHC, May 16, 1995 (increase in aggression, Luvox decreased to 25 mg, "this is obviously a complicated case"); my interview with Gene Deterling (with Curtis and medications, less is better than more).

Chapter 21: A New Voice, A New Frankness

For biographical details on Janalee Heinemann and her family, my sources are: *TGV,* November 1986, page 3 (Janalee's background in social work); Tomaseski-Heinemann, "A Parent's Point of View," Chapter 18 in *Mgt of PWS* 1st Ed., page 182 (Janalee raising three children on her own when she met Al and his children, Matt and Sarah), page 183 (Matt seemed relieved when the food was locked up); *TGV,* July 1984, page 9 (Al cried after seeing adolescents with PWS at his first national conference); Heinemann, "Growing Up with Prader-Willi Syndrome" (presentation at 2007 PWSA conference in Dallas) (Janalee Heinemann gave me a copy of this document) ("We came home [from the 1981 PWSA conference] and locked the refrigerator"); *TGV,* November 1986, page 3 (Janalee and Al started the first Missouri chapter in 1982).

For Janalee's writings on PWS, my sources are: *TGV,* November 1982, page 6 (announcing a book written by Janalee and Sarah); Janalee, "Understanding Chronic Grief," *TGV,* July 1984, page 9; Tomaseski-Heinemann, "A Parent's Point of View," Chapter 18 in *Mgt of PWS* 1st Ed.

For the changes in the leadership of PWSA, my sources are: *TGV,* July 1986, page 1 (Janalee elected to PWSA board);

my interview with Gene and Fausta Deterling (impressed with Janalee's leadership abilities, Sam being a little too anxious and dominating conversation led people to want another president, Marge may have been a little domineering); my interview with Sam Beltran (Janalee was dynamic and a good leader, he walked out of the board meeting when he lost support, he and Marge had rubbed several people the wrong way); my interview with Lota Mitchell (Sam stormed out of the board meeting); *TGV,* September 1990 page 12 (Sam fired himself); *TGV,* May 1991, page 1 (Janalee new president of PWSA); *TGV,* August 1991, page 11 (Marge resigned as executive director); my interview with Marge Wett (board was pushing for more professional printing but Marge wanted to keep doing it the old, affordable way); *TGV,* September 1992, page 8 (around three hundred members when Marge became executive director in 1980); *TGV,* September 1990, page 2 (membership is 1,583); *TGV,* March 1981, page 8 (financial report for 1980); *TGV,* January 1990, page 2 (planned expenses for 1990 of $105,000); *TGV,* September 1990, page 2 (twenty-six group homes for PWS now).

Chapter 22: A Medicine for PWS

All of the biographical details on Sam Beltran come from my interview with him. For Sam's involvement with growth hormone, the sources are my interview with Sam (chief of pediatrics at Stanford tried to discourage him and finally referred him to Ron Rosenfeld); my interview with Ron Rosenfeld (Sam

Beltran convinced him to try Sarah on GH for a year, Sarah was happy and proud of the good results); *TGV,* September 1983, page 9 (Sam's daughter grew four inches after one year on GH and another inch in the next three months); my interview with Phillip Lee (GH shots were initially intramuscular and painful).

For Phillip Lee and his involvement with PWS and GH, most of the details come from my interview with him. Other sources: Lee, "Growth Hormone Treatment of Short Stature in Prader-Willi Syndrome," *Journal of Pediatric Endocrinology* 2(1):31–34 (1987) (treating four patients with PWS); Lee, "Body Composition Studies in Prader-Willi Syndrome: Effects of Growth Hormone Therapy," in *Human Body Composition* (New York: Plenum Press, 1993), pages 201–205.

For Moris Angulo and Barbara Whitman, most of the details come from my interviews with them. Other sources: December 20, 2015 email from Angulo (started giving GH to patients with PWS in mid-1980s); Angulo, "Pituitary Evaluation and Growth Hormone Treatment in Prader-Willi Syndrome," *Journal of Pediatric Endocrinology* 4:167–173 (1991); Angulo, "Growth Hormone Secretion and Effects of Growth Hormone Therapy on Growth Velocity and Weight Gain in Children with Prader-Willi Syndrome," *Journal of Pediatric Endocrinology and Metabolism* 9:393–400 (1996).

For other reports on GH in PWS, and the controversy about whether GH should be given to people with PWS, the sources are: Eiholzer, "Treatment with Human Growth Hormone in Patients with Prader-Labhart-Willi Syndrome

Reduces Body Fat and Increases Muscle Mass and Physical Performance," *European Journal of Pediatrics* 157:368–377 (1998); *TGV,* October 1996, insert "Policy Statement: GH Treatment and Prader-Willi Syndrome"; Lindgren, "Growth Hormone Treatment of Children with Prader-Willi Syndrome Affects Linear Growth and Body Composition Favourably," *Acta Paediatrica* 87(1):28–31 (January 1998) (controlled study); Hauffa, "One-Year Results of Growth Hormone Treatment of Short Stature in Prader-Willi Syndrome," *Acta Paediatrica* (suppl) 423:63–65 (1997) (controlled study); Carrel, "Growth Hormone Improves Body Composition, Fat Utilization, Physical Strength and Agility, and Growth in Prader-Willi Syndrome: A Controlled Study," *The Journal of Pediatrics* 134(2):215–221 (February 1999); *TGV,* July 1999, page 10 (Hanchett on parents who stopped GH because of concerns about behavior management); *TGV,* October 1996, page 7 (Hanchett on a parent who felt her child would be treated more gently if shorter, and another who feared she could no longer control her son's behavior if he exceeded her in height); *TGV,* June 2000, page 1 (mother of two-year-old had studied GH carefully and started it when her child with PWS was seven months old, FDA approved Pharmacia's GH in PWS); *TGV,* June 2000, page 5 (PWS board of consultants chaired by Lee).

For the sudden death controversy, the main source is my interview with Urs Eiholzer, supplemented by an email from him dated November 3, 2015 (he had treated more than ten very young children with PWS with GH, Prader pointed out Eiholzer had done a study showing GH deficiency was innate in PWS). Other sources: Eiholzer, "Fatal Outcome of Sleep Apnoea in PWS during the Initial Phase of Growth Hormone Treatment," *Hormone Research* 58(suppl 3):24–26 (2002) (boy); Nordmann and Eiholzer, "Sudden Death of an Infant with Prader-Willi Syndrome—Not a Unique Case?," *Biology of the Neonate* 82:139–141 (2002); Eiholzer, "Deaths in Children with Prader-Willi Syndrome: A Contribution to the Debate about the Safety of Growth Hormone Treatment in Children with PWS," *Hormone Research* 63:33–39 (2005), page 38 (GH therapy can cause initial fluid retention and exacerbate growth of tonsils); Heinemann, "Concerns about Addressing Deaths and the Relationship to Growth Hormone," *TGV,* July 2003, page 3 (PWSA receiving emails and calls of concern, Matt's experience with GH, fear that doctors would stop prescribing GH, Pfizer's new label); October 21, 2015 email from Janalee Heinemann to John Storr (reaction by some countries to GH controversy); Eisen, "Mexico Conference 2003: It All Started with Jacobus," *TGV,* May 2004, page 6 (GH not an alternative given the economics of Mexico).

Chapter 23: Lessons of Genetics

Sources for the hope and reality of further genetic break-throughs: *TGV,* November 1988, page 3 (researcher at conference said gene therapy was "certainly a possibility in the next ten years"); *TGV,* March 1990, page 4 (quoting doctor who expected "successful treatment of many genetic disorders" in the 1990s); *TGV,* January 1992, page 6 (Janalee: "We are greatly encouraged by the many news articles regarding the progress in the field of genetics"); Buiting and Horsthemke, "Molecular Genetic Findings in PWS," Chapter 3 in *Mgt of PWS*, 3rd Ed (2006), pages 63–64 (paternally expressed genes in Prader-Willi imprinted region are MKRN3, MAGEL2, NDN and SNURF-SNRPN); Sutcliffe and Beaudet, "Deletions of a Differentially Methylated CpG Island at the SNRPN Gene Define a Putative Imprinting Control Region," *Nature Genetics* 8:52–58 (September 1994); Cattanach, "A Candidate Mouse Model for Prader-Willi Syndrome which Shows an Absence of *Snrpn* Expression," *Nature Genetics* 2:270-274 (December 1992); Driscoll, "Recent Advances in the Research and Treatment of Obesity: How They Relate to the Prader-Willi Syndrome," *TGV*, July 1998, page 6 (three different research groups made PWS mouse models but all died at a young age), page 7 (researchers looking for PWS-like patients with a mutation in one of the imprinted PWS-region genes); Nicholls, "New Insights Reveal Complex Mechanisms Involved in Genomic Imprinting," *American Journal of Human Genetics* 54:733–740 (1994), page 735 (important to find PWS-like patients with mutation in one PWS-region gene); Nicholls and Cassidy, "'Obese' Gene News Reports Overstated... (But Will Lead to Better Understanding of Obesity in General)," *TGV*, February 1995, page 5 (bold claim); Driscoll, "Mouse Models of PWS—How Similar to PWS Are They and What Will We Learn From Them?," *TGV*, July 2004, page 7 (abstract of presentation at International PWS conference in New Zealand: "no one has created a mouse model that closely resembles all the major clinical features of PWS, particularly the obesity and hyperphagia"); my interview with Nicholls (mouse not a great model for PWS because does not model the hyperphagia and obesity). Sources showing scientists' differing views on which genes cause PWS: *compare* my interview with Nicholls (he thought multiple genes contributed to PWS) *with* my interview with Beaudet (he thought 80 percent of PWS phenotype was from SNORD116 with other bits from NDN, MAGEL2 region).

Sources for why the deletion causing PWS keeps occurring in humans: Amos-Landgraf and Nicholls, "Chromosome Breakage in the Prader-Willi and Angelman Syndromes Involves Recombination between Large, Transcribed Repeats at Proximal and Distal Breakpoints," *American Journal of Human Genetics* 65:370–386 (1999); Christian and Ledbetter, "Large Genomic Duplicons Map to Sites of Instability in the Prader-Willi/Angelman Syndrome Chromosome Region (15q11-q13)," *Human Molecular Genetics* 8(6):1025–1037 (1999); en.wikipedia.org/w/index.php?title=Semen_analysis&oldid=620971176 (retrieved August 12, 2014) (typical male produces 20 million to 40 million sperm per ml, and typical volume of ejaculate is 1 to 6.5 ml, meaning approximately 100 million sperm per ejaculation on average); Butler, "Genomic Imprinting Disorders in Humans: A Mini-Review," *Journal of Assisted Reproduction and Genetics* 26:477–486 (2009), page 479 (PWS estimated to occur in 1 in 15,000 individuals; 70 percent of PWS cases are caused by deletion); "simple math": (.000067 births are PWS) × (.7 of PWS births caused by deletion) × 100,000,000 sperm = 4,690 sperm causing PWS.

Sources for why maternal UPD of chromosome 15 occurs: Cassidy, "Trisomy 15 with Loss of the Paternal 15 as a Cause of Prader-Willi Syndrome Due to Maternal Disomy," *American Journal of Human Genetics* 51:701–708 (1992); mosaicism.cfri. ca/specific/trisomy15.htm (retrieved October 21, 2015) ("complete trisomy 15 is a lethal abnormality"); my interview with Nicholls (same); Hall, "Genomic Imprinting: Review and Relevance to Human Diseases," *American Journal of Human Genetics* 46:857–873 (1990), page 860 (description of trisomy rescue without using the term); Carey, "Introductory Comments— Special Section: Prader-Willi Syndrome," *American Journal of Medical Genetics*, Part A, 143A:413–414 (2007) (using the term "trisomy rescue" in regard to UPD in PWS); my interview with Nicholls ("You or I may have started out as trisomy 15, but if we lost one of our two maternals, we're okay now."); Pollack, "Seeking Clues to Obesity in Rare Hunger Disorder," *The New York Times*, January 14, 2014 (PWSA knows of 8,000 Americans with PWS); Butler, "Genomic Imprinting Disorders in Humans: A Mini-Review," *Journal of Assisted Reproduction and Genetics* 26:477–486 (2009), page 479 (25 percent of PWS cases are caused by UPD); Cassidy, "Genetics of Prader-Willi Syndrome," Chapter 2 in *Mgt of PWS*, 2nd Ed., page 23 (Down syndrome is caused by trisomy 21), page 24 (as in Down syndrome, mothers of children with UPD PWS tend to be older).

Parents who found ways to make stories out of genetics: Ali Shenk, "Ask The Parents II," *TGV*, November 2006, page 6 (our "limited edition" baby); Jennifer Rinkenberger, "Thoughts on Healing," *TGV*, July 2009, page 12 (No thanks, Mr. Sperm).

Sources for evolutionary theorists on imprinting in general: Tilghman, "The Sins of the Fathers and Mothers:

Genomic Imprinting in Mammalian Development," *Cell* 96:185–193 (January 22, 1999), page 185 ("genetic paradox" of turning off a good copy of a gene); Wilkins and Haig, "What Good is Genomic Imprinting: The Function of Parent-Specific Gene Expression," *Nature Reviews: Genetics* 4:1–10 (May 2003), page 1 ("evolutionary puzzle"), page 4 (the theory is best known as the conflict theory although the authors prefer kinship theory); Nicholls, "Genetic Abnormalities in Prader-Willi Syndrome and Lessons from Mouse Models," *Acta Paediatrica* (suppl) 433:99–104 (1999), page 103 (Haig's theory is the best-supported theory for evolution of imprinting); Ubeda, "Evolution of Genomic Imprinting with Biparental Care: Implications for Prader-Willi and Angelman Syndromes," *PLoS Biology* 6(8) e208 (August 2008), page 1678 (kinship theory [aka conflict theory] "is currently the most widely accepted"); Haig and Westoby, "Parent-Specific Gene Expression and the Triploid Endosperm," *The American Naturalist* 134(1):147–155 (July 1989), page 149 (if females sometimes have offspring with other males, then the paternal genes will favor more resource acquisition from the mother); Haig, "Alice in Wonderland," *Genomic Imprinting and Kinship* (New Brunswick, NJ: Rutgers University Press, 2002), page 46 ("Maternal and paternal genes of an embryo have a large overlap of interests in ensuring a successful outcome of development").

Sources on evolutionary theories of Prader-Willi syndrome: Haig, "Conflicting Messages: Genomic Imprinting and Internal Communication," Chapter 12 in *Sociobiology of Communication*

(Oxford University Press, 2008), pages 219–220 (rare mishaps give hint of what genes normally do, discussion of PWS); Haig, "Prader-Willi Syndrome and the Evolution of Human Childhood," *American Journal of Human Biology* 15:320–329 (2003); Haig, "Genomic Imprinting and the Evolutionary Psychology of Human Kinship," *Proceedings of the National Academy of Sciences* 108(suppl 2):10878–10885 (2011), page 10880 (PWS babies' poor suckling, weak cry, and excessive sleepiness suggest paternal genes that promote suckling, strength of cry, and wakefulness).

Sources for the importance of PWS to researchers: Esteller, "The Necessity of a Human Epigenome Project," *Carcinogenesis* 27(6):1121–1125 (2006), page 1123 (abnormal methylation in cancer is same mechanism as abnormal methylation in PWS and Angelman, autoimmune disorders also have massive hypomethylation); Carey, "Introductory Comments—Special Section: Prader-Willi Syndrome," *American Journal of Medical Genetics*, Part A, 143A:413–414 (2007) (listing all the new concepts in medical genetics that PWS has played a role in).

Chapter 24: Curtis Finds a New Bottom

For Curtis's difficulties at Laura Baker, the main sources are my interviews with Bruce Jensen and Deana Antley. Other sources: my interviews with Gene and Fausta (new woman came in who claimed she knew about PWS but made everything worse, Curtis placed with non-PWS clients and expected to eat just his small share, some Laura Baker staff lacked the education and smarts to deal with PWS clients, staff having to hold a screaming Curtis back when Gene and Fausta left); my interviews with Curtis (some of the Laura Baker staffers did or said mean things).

For Curtis's psychiatric issues prior to hospitalization: SCCHC, October 29, 1998 report (discontinued Luvox for Celexa, a new SSRI); SCCHC, May 21, 1998 report (suicidal talk, said he'd been under stress but couldn't say why); SCCHC, April 13, 1999 report (Curtis refused Buspar, Kern talked to him about herbals); SCCHC, August 24, 1999 report (taking valerian); Allina Health file on Curtis Deterling (hereafter "Allina") December 1, 1999 risk management report (ax, throwing things); SCCHC, February 29, 2000 report (significantly more aggressive, refused appointments, wanted to be off Celexa); Allina, March 9, 2000 admission form to Abbot Northwestern (discontinued Celexa March 1); Allina, March 10, 2000 exam by Knudson (Curtis's violence in prior week).

For Curtis's first hospitalization at Abbott Northwestern: Allina, March 9, 2000 ambulance report (Curtis threatening and combative that morning, staff called 911, DeeDee accompanied Curtis); Allina, March 9, 2000 Northfield emergency room report (took five or six workers to restrain him at Laura Baker that morning); Allina, March 9, 2000 note (Curtis to be transferred to Abbott Northwestern); my interview with Antley (went with Curtis to hospital on day he was transferred to Abbott Northwestern); Allina, March 9, 2000 Northfield emergency room report (seventy-two-hour hold, combative when blood pressure was attempted); Allina, March 9, 2000 Northfield progress report (Curtis refused to take any medication); Allina, March 9, 2000 Northfield ambulance report (taking him to Abbott Northwestern); Allina, March 9, 2000 progress report (Curtis to be placed at Abbott station 47 [mental health unit]); en.wikipedia.org/w/index.php?title=Abbott_Northwestern_Hospital&oldid=638850905 (retrieved December 30, 2014) (Abbott Northwestern is a large teaching and specialty hospital in Minnesota); Allina, March 9, 2000 restraint/seclusion report (first day at the hospital); Allina, March 10, 2000 restraint/seclusion report (morning problems); Allina, March 10, 2000 report by Knudson (Curtis was evasive and stressed, plan was for Celexa and Neurontin); en.wikipedia.org/w/index.php?title=Gabapentin&oldid=639349786 (retrieved December 30, 2014) (Gabapentin aka Neurontin); Allina, March 13, Knudson entry (stopped Celexa and increased Neurontin because of manic symptoms); Allina, March 12, 2000 report (Curtis "organizing" the breakfast cart); Allina, March 13, 2000 report (Curtis drinking another patient's soda); Allina, March 13, 2000 report (Curtis told nurse "later" when she wanted to weigh him); Allina, March 13, 2000 report ("body odor extreme"); Allina, March 14, 2000 report (finally took shower); Allina, March 14, 2000 clinical data record (weighed 172); Allina, March 13, 2000 report (interrupts constantly); Allina, March 12, 2000 report (needs repeated limits); Allina, March 14, 2000 report (confronted about humor at others' expense); Allina, March 9, 2000 progress record (Fausta calling in with information on Haldol); Allina, March 9, 2000 physician's orders (prescribing Haldol and then canceling it); Allina, March 10, 2000 restraint/

seclusion report (parents visited, brought toy, encouraged taking medications); Allina, March 14, 2000 physician's orders (parents may bring cat for visit); Allina, March 15, 2000 report (angry and crying when he heard Laura Baker would reduce his calories to 1,200); Allina, March 15, 2000 report (Curtis refused to leave, deal worked out over 1,200 calorie diet).

For Curtis's second hospitalization at Abbott Northwestern: Allina, April 10, 2000 report by Knudson (Curtis saying Gene and Fausta were not his real parents, barricaded in his room Saturday night, fearful of hairy monster, walked away from Laura Baker); Allina April 9, 2000 Abbott Northwestern intake papers (Dukes of Hazzard being his real parents, plan to go to California); my interview with Fausta Deterling (Curtis found by staffer and brought back to Laura Baker); Allina, April 9, 2000 ambulance report (intent to show he wasn't crazy, adding "E-O" to end of each word); my interview with Antley (Curtis's deterioration the worst thing she'd ever seen); Allina, April 9, 2000 intake interview (delusional yet articulate); Allina, April 10, 2000 report by Knudson (schizoaffective disorder, Risperdal and Depakote); www.webmd.com/drugs/2/drug-1788/depakote-oral/details (retrieved October 22, 2015); Allina, April 10, 2000 nursing report (yelling at big hairy monster); Allina, April 11, 2000 nursing report (yelling, running in halls, rolling around, removing clothes); Allina, April 12, 2000 nursing report (taking clothes off, toilet overflowing, dive into ping pong table); Allina, April 13, 2000 report (kept clothes on, attended some groups for short periods, but also spoke of hairy monster); Allina, April 13, 2000 report (calm during parents' visit but also pounded on doors, urinated on floor); Allina, April 14, 2000 physician's note (adding Zyprexa, Ativan); en.wikipedia.org/w/index.php?title=Ol anzapine&oldid=680794210 (retrieved October 22, 2015) (Zyprexa); en.wikipedia.org/w/index.php?title=Lorazepam &oldid=686184545 (retrieved October 22, 2015) (Ativan); Allina, April 19, 2000 Knudson report (Curtis improved on new medication regimen); Allina, April 18, 2000 report (Curtis pleasant and cooperative); Allina, April 17, 2000 physician's note (Curtis said the hairy monster wasn't real); Allina, April 15, 16, and 18 reports, 2000 (parents visited); Allina, April 17, 2000 physician's note (Gene said Celexa was helpful in the past); Allina, April 19, 2000 Knudson report (Celexa was added late during the hospital stay); Allina, April 18, 2000 social worker's note (Curtis has strong family support); Allina, April 19, 2000 note (Curtis excited to be discharged, pleasant).

Chapter 25: The Last Stop

For Marty McGraw, the source is my interview with him.

For Curtis moving into Marty's group home in Underwood, the sources are: Laura Baker file on Curtis (Curtis left Laura Baker on March 30, 2001, weighed 181); my interview with Kevin Tobias (Curtis's black leather outfit the day he started at AME house in Underwood, rough start, phone calls to parents, Gene and Fausta taking Curtis's word over staff at times, better after Marty communicated with them); my interview with Gene Deterling (Curtis's room at Laura Baker very messy, cleaning it out); my interview with Jeb Sawyer (feared Curtis had weapons in his closet at Laura Baker, but saving grace was that the room was so profoundly messy); my interview with Marty McGraw (letter he sent the Deterlings and his conversation with Fausta); my interview with Gene and Fausta (reaction to Marty's letter).

For Curtis's experiences at Underwood, the first of Marty's homes that he lived in, my sources are mostly from the files of Marty's company, AME. In particular: AME, May 2004 annual (Curtis weighed 163 on May 3); AME, December psychological and medical review (fewer disruptive behaviors in 2003, dropped from Opportunity Partners as of March 2003, not consistently exercising, very slow at completing hygiene activities); my interview with Sandy Singer (female housemate at AME dying suddenly of stomach necrosis); my interview with Curtis (Kathy Olson was the housemate at Underwood who died); my interview with Gene and Fausta Deterling (Kathy Olson's sudden death from stomach rupture); AME, December 2003 psychological and medical review (in spring Curtis and housemate moved to Plymouth home); my interview with Kevin Tobias (death of female housemate prompted move to Plymouth home, untactful response to Kathy Olson's death, asking about her movies).

For Curtis's experiences at Plymouth: AME, May 2004 annual (Curtis weighed 144 on April 4); AME, December 2004 psychological and medical review (difficulty with routines and worksite, food seeking, first appointment with Hardrict, tapered Depakote and increased Celexa); AME, December 2004 psychological and medical review (Hardrict started Curtis on Seroquel in March 2005); AME, April 29, 2005 functional review (new data collection plan); AME, April 29, 2005 Minnesota Department of Human Services program (program recommendations, including reinforcers); my interview with Kevin Tobias (medications and new behavior plan: nearly a 180-degree change in Curtis, staff learned to not take it personally when Curtis got verbally abusive and to engage with questions, Kevin joined AME two weeks before the Underwood home opened April 1, 2001, rewards for not skin picking, actually got Curtis to stop picking on regular basis); AME, December 2005 psychological and medical review (Hardrict shocked at behavior improvement at September 28, 2005 appointment); AME, May 2007 annual (returned to the YMCA in August 2006, daily routines "markedly improved," behavior calmer and attitude more flexible, raising the bar by working on tendencies to try to go over the heads of staff and to use racial slurs); AME, May 2006 annual (details of social stories, and of tracking racial slurs); AME, October 2011 progress notes (incident with incense vendor); AME, progress notes February 2012 (incident with bank teller); AME, July 2008 annual (lost job collating brochures due to bleeding from picking); AME, July 2012 progress notes (program coordinator warned Curtis that he couldn't go out if he kept picking).

For the sweeter side of Curtis's personality: my interview with Kevin Tobias (Curtis liked to pick up trash along 36th

Avenue for Mother Earth, Curtis focused on his girlfriend on her birthday and on Valentine's Day, once sang her a song, "we're a laughing household," picking out some horrible movie and laughing at it, doing better at work, back at the job collating brochures, appropriate reaction in 2010 to death of an AME client and comforted the mother); AME, August 2012 progress notes (picked up trash by 36th Ave on August 11); AME, December 2012 progress notes (shoveled house driveway, then neighbor's driveway on December 9); AME, April 2012 progress notes (visiting the humane society); AME, May 2011 to April 2012 progress review (volunteering for picnic, getting Christmas gifts); my interview with Curtis (his plans with his girlfriend); AME, April 2011 progress notes (housemates having fun laughing at horror film on April 9); AME, November 2012 progress notes (Curtis thankful for great family and happy to be living at AME); AME, December 2011 progress notes (toasting Marty at Christmas party); AME, November 2012 progress notes (took sauce packets at movie theater on December 2).

Postscript

Sources for Zellweger and Prader: Wiedemann, "Hans-Ulrich Zellweger (1909–1990)," *European Journal of Pediatrics*, 150:451 (1991) (eighty years old at death); my interview with James Hanson (Zellweger's suicide); Zachmann, "Andrea Prader 1919–2001," *Hormone Research* 56:205–207 (2002).

Made in the USA
San Bernardino, CA
31 August 2016